THE

Basic·Basics·

DIABETES

HANDBOOK

THE
Basic Basics

DIABETES

HANDBOOK

JANE FRANK

GRUB STREET · LONDON

ACKNOWLEDGEMENTS

Without all the help I was given by three groups of people this book would never have been written. First the people with diabetes who kindly agreed to be interviewed: David, Dorothea, Gay, Henrietta, Jean, Laura, Mike and Rona. Together they helped me to be aware of the role that diabetes plays in people's lives, and they gave me a better understanding of the disease. Henrietta, in particular, has not only given me insights into the physical implications of diabetes but has also demonstrated that, while the illness can sometimes be a trial, it can also be spiritually enriching.

The second and indispensable group of people consists of all those, either diabetics or nutritionists, and sometimes both, who tested and commented on the recipes. Special thanks go to Alexandra Aitken, Lynn Alford-Burow, Marion Billingham, Kay Clarke, Josie Cowgill, Fiona McDonald Joyce, Rona MacInnes, Linda Marais, Nicola Phipps and Jake, Sara Shakespeare, Coreen Tucker, David Wallace and Kasumi Hatazawa, Penny Williams and Craig Brown, and Liz Wright. Not only did they correct me where I went wrong, and give me honest opinions about the taste and appearance of my creations, but they also ensured that all the recipes went through a robust testing process, and are therefore, if not foolproof, at least as unambiguous as I could make them.

For going through my facts with a fine-toothed comb and correcting my tendency to obscurity, my heartfelt thanks go to my husband John and to my old colleague Mike Frazer. And finally, I owe a huge debt of gratitude to Gay Patton, a diabetes nurse and educator and a diabetic herself, who read through the introduction very carefully and made many constructive comments. Thank you all.

First published in 2004 by
Grub Street
4 Rainham Close
London
SW11 6SS
Email: food@grubstreet.co.uk
www.grubstreet.co.uk

A CIP record for this book is available from the British Library

ISBN 1 904010 75 X

Typeset by Pearl Graphics, Hemel Hempstead
Printed and bound in Great Britain by Biddles Ltd, King's Lynn

CONTENTS

INTRODUCTION

It is neither alarmist nor an exaggeration to say that we are in the midst of an epidemic of diabetes in the Western world, but simply a statement of fact. In 2002 it was estimated that there were 2.5 million people in the UK with diabetes, and nearly 20 million in the USA[1]. It is appearing increasingly in the developing world too, especially in Asian countries such as Korea and Taiwan and in urban populations in India and Pakistan[2]. The number of people with diabetes globally is currently estimated at 194 million, and that number is predicted to rise to 366 million in 2030, according to the International Diabetes Federation and World Health Organisation statistics.

Why is diabetes on the increase? Epidemiologists say that it is due to our more and more sedentary life style, the overabundance of processed foods and, more specifically in Europe and America, an ageing population.[3] Diabetes is associated with obesity, but recent findings indicate that the diabetes epidemic will continue even if levels of obesity remain constant. But because obesity continues to rise, it is likely that the predictions for diabetes are actually an underestimate[4].

Diabetes research has made enormous progress over the last few years, and a much greater understanding of the disease, its causes and risk factors, has developed. However, some of the advice given to people with diabetes has not always kept pace with the research. This book aims to fill that gap. The information and the recipes it contains are based on the latest research and on informed medical opinion. However, I hope the recipes are simple enough for anyone to cook. This book is intended both for people with diabetes, whether they have been newly diagnosed or whether they are old hands, and also for those people who are aware of the risks of diabetes and who wish to minimise those risks by modifying their diet.

WHAT IS DIABETES?

Put simply, diabetes is a condition in which there is too much glucose (sugar) in the blood. This glucose comes from the carbohydrate foods in our diet, and is the principal source of energy for the muscles and the brain. The level of blood glucose is normally strictly regulated by two hormones called insulin and glucagon, secreted by the pancreas, at between 80-100mg/dl (milligrams per decilitre of blood) when the stomach is empty, and up to 140mg/dl just after a meal. Working in tandem, the function of insulin is to lower blood glucose whilst that of glucagon is to raise it. In diabetes, this mechanism fails to work, and the blood glucose level is abnormally high. This could be either because the pancreas makes too little or no insulin, or because the cells become resistant to insulin and fail to respond to its message.

SIGNS AND SYMPTOMS

The first effect of high blood glucose levels, above 160-180mg/dl, is that glucose passes into the urine because it can't get into the cells where it is needed. This glucose makes the urine of a person with undiagnosed diabetes sweet, hence the name 'diabetes mellitus' – 'mellitus' deriving from the Greek word for honey. In response to these high levels of glucose, the kidneys excrete more fluid in an attempt to dilute the urine. This results in the need to pass urine more frequently (polyuria), which, in turn, causes extreme thirst (polydipsia). The excessive fluid loss often causes the patient to lose weight, which may make them feel very hungry (polyphagia). Polyuria, polydipsia and polyphagia are the three classic symptoms of diabetes. Other symptoms include extreme fatigue, blurred vision, nausea and tingling or numbness in the hands and feet. Frequent or recurring infections and slow wound healing are also signs of undiagnosed diabetes.

A simple fasting plasma glucose test can confirm whether or not you have diabetes. The test is given in a lab or at the GP's surgery, usually in the morning, after fasting since the previous evening. If the fasting plasma glucose level is 120 mg/dl or higher, even after not eating for eight hours, it usually means that the person has diabetes.

Fasting serum insulin levels are often tested as well. They should be under 10 mIU/ml (milli-international units per millilitre) and ideally under 5 mIU/ml. High insulin levels after an 8 hour fast mean that the cells are resistant to insulin. Any fasting insulin level over 10 mIU/ml is a major problem and is a risk factor for diabetes.

TYPES OF DIABETES

There are two main types of diabetes mellitus: Type 1 and Type 2. About 5% of people with diabetes have Type 1, while the remainder are Type 2. The two types are very different from each other, although management of both conditions is broadly similar.

Type 1 or Insulin-Dependent Diabetes Mellitus (IDDM)

In this type, which used to be called juvenile diabetes to distinguish it from the later-onset Type 2, the symptoms listed above begin suddenly and must receive immediate medical attention. If it is not recognised immediately, a condition called diabetic ketoacidosis (DKA) may result. Although there is a lot of glucose in the blood, the cells can't use it because there is no insulin. The body interprets this as starvation, and so it uses fat as a source of energy instead. The breakdown of fat cells results in the formation of ketones, strong acid compounds that make the blood more acid (ketoacidosis). The acid/alkaline balance of the blood (the pH), like the blood sugar level, is normally kept within strict limits (a pH of 7.35-7.45) by various mechanisms, one of which is the exhalation of carbon dioxide. Breathing out reduces the level of acid in the blood, so a person going through diabetic ketoacidosis will breathe deeply and rapidly in an attempt to make the blood less acid. The exhaled acid on such a person's breath smells like pear drops. Without treatment, diabetic ketoacidosis can result in coma and eventually death. People with established Type 1 diabetes can develop ketoacidosis if they miss an insulin injection or become stressed by an infection, an accident, or a serious medical condition.

Type 1 diabetes is sometimes further classified into three subtypes:

Immune-mediated diabetes (Type 1A). This form results from auto-immune destruction of the beta cells of the pancreas. Interestingly, about 5% of people with auto-immune diabetes also have coeliac disease (an auto-immune disorder of digestive tract that is triggered by gluten in wheat and other grains, and which leads to a malabsorption of all nutrients, primarily of fat).

Idiopathic diabetes (Type 1B). Some forms of Type 1 diabetes have no known cause. Some diabetics have permanent insulin deficiency and are prone to ketoacidosis but have no evidence of auto-immunity. This form of diabetes is strongly inherited and is more common in people of African or Asian heritage.

Latent Auto-immune Diabetes in Adults (or Slow Onset Type 1, LADA or Type 1.5). This is Type 1 diabetes appearing in adulthood (over the age of 30). These patients do not immediately require insulin for treatment, are often not overweight, and have little or no resistance to insulin. They are often diagnosed as Type 2 because they are older and will initially respond to diabetes medications because they have adequate insulin production.[5] One major benefit to this type is that when their blood sugars are controlled, people with Type 1.5 usually do not have the high risk for heart problems more often found with the high cholesterol and blood pressure seen in true Type 2 diabetes.

DAVID

David is a very unusual Type 1 diabetic, in that he was not diagnosed until the age of 36, so he could more properly be said to have Latent Autoimmune Diabetes in Adults (LADA, also known as Type 1.5). He was put onto Metformin initially, but after a while this appeared not to be working. This is not surprising as the primary action of this drug is to overcome insulin resistance, whereas David's problem was not insulin resistance so much as poor insulin production. Eventually he was put on insulin therapy, and he now takes two types – Humalog at meal times, and a new long-lasting insulin called Lantus at night. The latter is supposed to last for 24 hours, but in practice David finds that it is not as beneficial as he had hoped, and often doesn't last long enough.

David describes himself as a 'foodie' in that he enjoys his food and is not prepared to deprive himself of the pleasures of the table. Typically for a person with LADA, he is not overweight. When first diagnosed with diabetes, he consulted a dietician, but found that the advice he was given was basic, old-fashioned and unsympathetic to his lifestyle. The emphasis was on processed foods such as baked beans, but David would never consider eating this sort of food. He did, however, broadly follow the recommended diet for the first two or three years, and then, unwilling to let his diabetes take over his life, he started 'flouting the rules'. For ten years his blood glucose levels were reasonably well-controlled, but they are now higher than they should be – typically 8-15 mmol/L, though he is not sure why. He has quite a stressful job, and it could be that this is a contributory factor. He exercises twice a week, and although he is well aware that exercising more frequently would help to moderate his blood sugar levels, David is a pragmatist and knows that he would not be able to find the time. At his 6-monthly checkups with the diabetes specialist, he has seen his HbA1C scores (see page 22) creeping up, and he is obviously concerned about this. The only real difference diabetes has made to his life is that he feels tired a lot of the time, but thankfully has none of the other complications of diabetes.

Breakfast for David, as for nearly all of my interviewees, often consists of porridge, as it is very good for moderating blood glucose levels. He also finds rice-based dishes help, though he is wary of relying overmuch on rice as it is a high-carbohydrate food. He gave up sugar in his tea and coffee long before he was diagnosed with diabetes, and he is lucky in that he doesn't have a particularly sweet tooth in any case. David feels that there isn't a lot of nutritional help for diabetics who really enjoy their food, so I hope he will find something of interest in this book.

Type 2 or Non-Insulin Dependent Diabetes Mellitus (NIDDM)

In Type 2, the same symptoms as those associated with Type 1 occur, but they progress gradually. They may not all be present, and sometimes people with Type 2 have no obvious symptoms at all, and are not even aware that they have diabetes. Such people may go undiagnosed for several years. As insulin deficiency progresses, symptoms may develop. Increased urination and thirst are mild at first and may gradually worsen over weeks or months. Ketoacidosis is rare. If the blood glucose level becomes very high – usually as the result of added stress such as an infection or drugs – the person may develop severe dehydration, which may lead to mental confusion, drowsiness or seizures.

One of the reasons Type 2 diabetes may remain undiagnosed for a long time is that many of its symptoms, such as increased urination, lack of energy, weight loss, skin infections, wounds that are slow to heal, or erectile dysfunction in men, are also complaints commonly associated with ageing. By the time a person is diagnosed, he or she may already be suffering from the complications of diabetes. Since untreated diabetes can cause blindness, kidney failure, heart disease and strokes, it is important to get it diagnosed and treated as soon as possible, particularly if you are in a high risk group.

MIKE

Mike was diagnosed as Type 2 less than a year before I interviewed him, but five years before that he had suspicions that he was already diabetic. At that time he went to the doctor with a lot of what he describes as 'little things' – skin irritation when he shaved, spots, sensitive skin, general lethargy – but there was never anything specific on which to pin these symptoms. On one of these visits to the doctor's surgery he saw a locum instead of his usual GP. The locum did a urine test which showed that Mike's urine glucose was very high. In the locum's opinion he was definitely diabetic, but on subsequent occasions his blood glucose, although high, was within normal limits. He was told he was glucose intolerant. The only dietary change he made at that time was to switch from sugar to sweeteners.

Mike's work involved a long commute on the motorway, and he was under a lot of pressure when he got into the office each day. By early 2003, he was feeling completely exhausted, and only kept himself going by eating chocolate and sweet snacks on the road. Then when he got home in the evenings he didn't feel like eating a proper meal. He was aware that his blood sugar levels were soaring, but he had almost ceased to care. Things came to a head one evening and he finally collapsed under the strain. He was diagnosed as diabetic after a glucose clearance test.

Mike keeps his diabetes under control by choosing low GI foods when possible. This is all right if he is at home or when he and his family go on self-catering holidays, but less easy when he has to stay in hotels on business. The only information he was given when he was first diagnosed was a pamphlet from Diabetes UK which advises consumption of bread, potatoes and pasta, suggests swapping sugar for sweeteners, and doesn't mention the GI at all. He discovered low GI eating by talking to a friend. When he mentioned the GI to his diabetes nurse, her response was 'Oh, it's 5 years since I looked at the glycaemic index'.

In Mike's opinion there is not enough quality help for people newly diagnosed with diabetes. He would like to see clear indications on food labels as to whether a food is good or bad for blood glucose control. An example is yoghurts, which are promoted as a healthy food, but which can be very high in sugar. He is still driving a lot, and comments that when you want a snack, the only options available in motorway services are sweet snacks such as chocolate, or fatty and salty snacks such as crisps. He makes sure he always has nuts and raisins in the glove-box of his car to help him avoid either of those unhealthy options.

Complications from Type 2 diabetes in adults can often be reduced or prevented with medicines, weight loss and exercise. However, it is uncertain what the prognosis is for those who start the disease in childhood rather than in adulthood, of whom there is an increasing number. Many doctors predict that complications will emerge in early adulthood.

Maturity-Onset Diabetes of the Young (MODY)
This is a hereditary form of diabetes usually occurring in people under the age of 25. MODY diabetes can often be controlled with diet or medication in the early stages. It differs from Type 2 diabetes in that patients have a defect in insulin secretion or glucose metabolism, and are not resistant to insulin. MODY accounts for about 2% of diabetes. Because MODY runs in families, it is useful for studying diabetes genes.

Gestational Diabetes
Gestational diabetes is a type of diabetes that occurs in pregnancy, and usually disappears after the baby is born. If not treated, it can cause serious problems for both the mother and the baby. Women belonging to high-risk ethnic groups, such as Afro-Caribbean, Hispanic, South or East Asian, are statistically more likely to get gestational diabetes. Other risk factors are overweight, age, family history of diabetes, having had gestational diabetes with a previous pregnancy, or having previously had a stillbirth or a very large baby.

Diabetes Insipidus
Despite the similar names, Diabetes Insipidus is not related to Diabetes Mellitus. It is a relatively rare condition that occurs when the kidneys are unable to conserve water, resulting in very diluted urine. Diabetes Insipidus can usually be managed by drinking adequate fluids and following a low-sodium diet.

THE CAUSES OF DIABETES

Experts continue to be at odds over the causes of diabetes, particularly of Type 1.

Type 1

There appears to be a genetic component in about 10% of people with Type 1. The most commonly accepted theory for its development in the other 90% is that viral infections, particularly those of the digestive system, cause the immune system to attack and destroy the islet cells of the pancreas where insulin is produced, rendering them unable to make insulin. Strongly implicated is the family of coxsackie viruses – polio-related viruses that cause upper respiratory infections. This is not a new theory – epidemiological studies in the 1960s, for example, showed that coxsackie outbreaks in various regions were followed by an increased incidence of diabetes.

Researchers in Finland have discovered that babies fed on cow's milk formula, particularly those with diabetic siblings, are five times more likely to develop Type 1 diabetes[6]. This may be because cow's milk contains insulin, and the babies may be making antibodies against the cow's insulin. These antibodies then go on to destroy the insulin-producing cells in the baby's pancreas. To support the theory that Type 1 is an auto-immune disease, 75% of people with diabetes have antibodies to their own pancreatic cells[7].

Type 2

In general, the risk of developing Type 2 diabetes rises with age, particularly after the age of 40. There is some hereditary component, so anyone who has a close relative with the disease might be considered at risk. Women who had diabetes when pregnant (gestational diabetes – see above) are at greater risk too. High blood pressure and membership of a high-risk ethnic group (such as Afro-Caribbean or Hispanic groups) also contribute to the risk. But the greatest risk factor is obesity. It is arguable whether obesity is the cause of diabetes or a symptom, along with diabetes itself, of pancreatic failure, but there is no doubt that obesity accompanies diabetes. Not all diabetics are overweight, but 90% of people who go on to develop Type 2 are overweight.

Unfortunately, Type 2 is now appearing in younger and younger people, especially in the United States but now also in the UK. Childhood Type 2 diabetes is characterised by obesity, high blood glucose levels and insulin resistance. The prevalence of obesity in UK children is increasing. Doctors blame the increasing diabetes trend on unhealthy diets and inactivity. Children with diabetes tend to be especially large for their age. Many also have a skin condition called acanthosis nigricans, dark patches around the neck and other skin folds, which is a sign of insulin resistance.

DOROTHEA

At a sprightly 82, Dorothea is the oldest of my interviewees and has had diabetes for thirty years. When she was about 50, she began to experience a terrible thirst, accompanied by itching all over her body. She went to the doctor and was swiftly diagnosed as having diabetes. This was a terrible shock to Dorothea. There was no diabetes in the family and she couldn't think where it had come from. She was started on tablets, and given help with managing her diet, but it quickly became apparent that she needed insulin. She was resistant to this at first, dreading having to cope with the injections, but eventually became used to it.

The recommended diet for diabetes thirty years ago appears to have made no distinction between refined and complex carbohydrates, and the Glycaemic Index hadn't been invented. By current standards the diet recommended to Dorothea seems designed to maintain rather high blood glucose, relying heavily on tea and biscuits between meals, toast for breakfast and a sandwich for lunch. Interestingly, before she had diabetes, Dorothea used to drink a lot of milk, but she was told to cut back on her milk consumption. She still largely follows the diet she was given back then, having her main meal in the evening consisting of a protein food, two potatoes and lots of vegetables, always with a small piece of fruit for dessert.

Two years ago Dorothea developed age-related macular degeneration, the effect of which she describes as like having a 'big black thing' in the centre of her vision. This makes it impossible to read, and she has to rely on a family member to read her mail for her. Drawing up her doses of insulin would be difficult too, without the help of the District Nurse, who visits three times a week to draw up the insulin for the following day.

Along with most other diabetics in this country, Dorothea was recently switched to the human insulin, and finds as a result that her blood sugar is much harder to control. She has always suffered from hypos (see page 17), for which she carries glucose tablets around with her. When she was on the porcine insulin, she says, she always knew when a hypo was coming on, as she would start yawning. But now, on the human insulin, she has no warning of hypos. She has also found that her blood sugar gets very low at bedtime, so she has started having a biscuit before going to bed to keep the blood sugar up during the night. This is typical of Dorothea's cheerful determination to cope with the vicissitudes of having diabetes.

RISK FACTORS FOR TYPE 2 DIABETES
Metabolic syndrome
Also known as Syndrome X or insulin resistance, this is a collection of symptoms that, taken together, predispose a person to

developing Type 2 diabetes. It can and usually does co-exist with the other risk factors.

To qualify for metabolic syndrome, a person must have at least three of the following characteristics:

- A waist measurement of more than 40"/102cm in men or 35"/89cm in women. In addition, a waist to hip ratio of more than 0.75 is considered a risk factor for diabetes
- High levels of triglycerides and LDL (low density lipoproteins) – the 'bad' cholesterol
- Low levels of HDL (high density lipoproteins) – the 'good' cholesterol. Low is considered to be less than 50 mmol/L (millimoles per litre) in women and less than 40 mmol/L in men.
- Blood pressure greater than 130/85mm Hg
- High levels of blood glucose
- Insulin resistance, which means that although the person may be producing enough insulin, the body cells are not heeding its message and taking up glucose as they should. The result is very often the coexistence of high blood glucose with excess circulating insulin.

Poor dietary choices
Most experts now agree that diets high in overall carbohydrates contribute to both diabetes and obesity by increasing the body's production of insulin. As long ago as 1935, Dr. H.D.C. Given pointed out the correlation between carbohydrate intake and diabetes[8]. More recently, Michel Montignac[9] has embraced a similar theory, now rapidly gaining credence, which states that obesity and Type 2 diabetes co-exist as symptoms of a pancreas that is not working properly and is producing too much insulin (hyper-insulinaemia). This surplus eventually causes insulin resistance. The reason the pancreas is producing too much insulin in the first place is a diet too high in refined carbohydrates and sugar.

To complicate the picture further, a diet low in fat, for example so-called 'heart-healthy' diets, can contribute to diabetes. If you remove fat, you are going to be left with too many carbohydrates. That will increase insulin, and anything that increases insulin over a long period of time is going to give you a higher risk for diabetes. So the danger of a so-called 'low fat' diet is not the low fat, but the high carbohydrate content.

There are good fats and bad fats, however. A diet high in hydrogenated fats – those fats found in processed foods – seems to increase the risk of Type 2 diabetes. As far back as the 1920s Dr. S. Sweeney produced reversible diabetes in his medical school students by feeding them a diet high in refined vegetable oils for 48 hours.

Three long term studies have recently shown that the foods most associated with a higher risk of Type 2 diabetes are: deep fried potatoes, white bread, white rice, crisps and fizzy drinks[10].

Chromium deficiency

A deficiency in the trace mineral chromium could be a contributory cause of Type 2 diabetes. Elevated insulin levels increase excretion of chromium, so people who receive insulin injections will tend to become deficient in chromium. Under normal circumstances, chromium works with insulin in allowing the cells to absorb and utilise glucose. A deficiency of chromium has been found to increase insulin requirements, so that a vicious cycle develops. Many Type 1 diabetics are also deficient in chromium.

Stress

Diabetes often develops after a stressful event such as a heart attack or car accident. Evidently emotional stress triggers hormonal responses. In particular insulin levels might fluctuate wildly – this is called post-traumatic dysinsulinism – with the result that blood glucose also fluctuates. This is in itself stressful and it is easy to see how poor insulin control can eventually result in mood swings, from depression to hypomania.[11]

HENRIETTA

Henrietta is the most unusual case of diabetes that I have come across, and is equally interesting to the many doctors who have cared for her over the years. Trauma accompanying the birth of her first child, now a strapping young man in his early twenties, triggered her diabetes. She lost 10 pints of blood during the Caesarian section, and the hospital was slow to get a transfusion in place. For three months after the birth, Henrietta was very weak – she had lost half her body weight, and was unable to feed her baby. Then the classic symptoms of diabetes began to appear – she became very thirsty and needed to urinate frequently, and her sight was affected. When she was diagnosed, she was found to need a very small dose of insulin indeed, and ever since has needed less than 10 units daily, sometimes in doses as small as half a unit. Henrietta is what is known as a brittle diabetic, in that her diabetes is particularly hard to manage. She used to have frequent hypos on the porcine insulin, but manages better with the human insulin. Occasionally she uses Humalog, but only in an emergency when she is given a high carbohydrate meal, perhaps at a dinner party.

Henrietta eats a very healthy diet. She doesn't avoid sugar completely, but is careful to balance high GI carbohydrates with low GI carbohydrates and protein. She long ago found that artificial sweeteners upset her digestive system, so she avoids these. She relies quite heavily on sugar-free muesli and porridge with which she will often have a banana. She cooks a lot of vegetarian dishes in her Aga, but is aware that roast peppers and parsnips, for example, are very high sugar, so she would never eat them on their own, but always with a low GI food or some protein. She does eat baked potatoes, but has discovered that the skins make her blood glucose leap up, so she usually leaves the skin.

Henrietta suffers from some of the complications of diabetes. Her legs were damaged during the birth of her first child, the skin on her legs is very thin and she bruises easily. Any wound on her legs is slow to heal. She always wears tubigrip bandages on her legs and makes sure to keep the blood circulating as much as possible by never sitting down for too long. Now she is starting to experience some neuropathy in her arms as well. She looks after her health carefully, walks everywhere and swims frequently. The worst thing, she finds, is that she is always tired, and has to make a conscious effort to rest as much as possible – about 10 hours a night – even if she is not asleep all that time.

Industrial air pollution

Dioxin intake by inhalation and/or ingestion has been revealed in published journals to be associated with an increased incidence of diabetes. Recent Israeli research has shown chronic exposure of fat or muscle cells to even low levels of free radicals produces insulin resistance and Type 2 diabetes[12]. In Sheffield the hospital admissions for diabetes were recorded per 1000 population as 4 in the city centre but as high as 11 in the eastern part of the city which is affected by pollution from dioxins emitted by the city incinerator and a castings plant.[13]

THE LONG-TERM IMPLICATIONS OF DIABETES

Diabetes is such an important issue because of the long-term effects of the disease. The complications of diabetes are serious. They include heart disease (2-4 times more likely in diabetics than in non-diabetics, high blood pressure (twice as common in diabetics), strokes (mortality rates from this disorder are three to six times higher in diabetics) and peripheral vascular disease (that is, diseases of the blood vessels outside the heart and brain, often a narrowing of vessels that carry blood to the leg muscles). There are several complications of diabetes that develop over time. These include damage to the retina of the eye (retinopathy), which can lead to impaired vision and even blindness. Other complications are damage to the blood vessels (angiopathy), the nervous system (neuropathy), and the kidneys (nephropathy). Studies show that keeping blood glucose levels as close to the normal, nondiabetic range as possible may help prevent, slow, or delay harmful effects to the eyes, kidneys, and nerves.

High blood glucose levels over an extended period result in glucose attaching to proteins until the proteins cease to function properly. This is called the glycosylation of proteins and, at the cellular level, is the ultimate cause of diabetic complications. Glycosylation reactions happen normally in the body, controlled by enzymes, but in diabetes the process is speeded up or uncontrolled. For example, cholesterol-carrying proteins that have been glycosylated are unable to bind to receptors that tell certain liver cells to stop manufacturing cholesterol. As a result, too much cholesterol is manufactured. For diabetics, the most significant glycosylation is that of haemoglobin, the molecule in our red blood cells which carries oxygen around the body. This glycosylation is measured by the HbA1C test (see page 22).

Glycosylated proteins eventually turn into Advanced Glycosylated End Products (AGEs) and their formation increases with the level and time that blood glucose is elevated. Glycosylation of the proteins in the lens of the eye can result in cataracts. AGEs also trigger the production of free radicals by the immune system. Free radicals are unstable molecules that can damage the DNA of cells. This increased level of free radical damage translates into high risk of developing many of the degenerative diseases. It has been found that people with metabolic syndrome, many of whom go on to develop Type 2 diabetes, have low antioxidant status[14]. It is therefore especially important that people at risk of diabetes protect themselves from free radical damage by eating a diet high in antioxidants, such as vitamins C and E, and by taking antioxidant supplements. (This is covered in more detail in the section on nutritional management.)

Hypoglycaemia

Hypoglycaemia means low blood sugar and is one of the effects of diabetes. People with diabetes unfortunately often experience hypoglycaemic episodes ('hypos') when their blood glucose is not under control. It may seem illogical that low blood sugar is the most dangerous effect of diabetes, which by its very nature is a disease of high blood sugar. However, hypoglycaemia arises if the person with diabetes injects too much insulin, or takes too high a dose of diabetes drugs. It can also occur if the person skips a meal or delays eating, drinks too much alcohol or exercises without eating beforehand. Low blood sugar, caused either by excess insulin or by lack of glucose from the diet, will lower the blood sugar too much, which causes the body to release adrenaline. The role of adrenaline is to mobilise energy stores and convert them into glucose. It also causes symptoms of nervous system stimulation and starves the brain of glucose, which can cause confusion and abnormal behaviour. Severe hypoglycaemia will result in coma and is eventually fatal. One diabetic I interviewed who has many years' experience of hypos, comments: 'I never know when I have a hypo coming on, and only realise when I become ludicrously depressed, clumsy, repetitive, exhausted. When I do realise what's happening, I have a large drink of orange juice. As I start to get better, usually after half an hour, I will test my blood and then have a small bowl of sugar-free muesli... You need to rest after a hypo – they are shattering to the system and need care and time to recover from.'

MEDICAL MANAGEMENT OF DIABETES

Before 1921, when insulin was first discovered, people with diabetes usually died, as there was no way to control their blood glucose levels. Today, people with Type 1 diabetes can manage their condition with insulin, and people with Type 2 diabetes either use medication to control their blood glucose, or manage the disease with diet and exercise alone. Some people with Type 2 also take insulin.

When a person is first diagnosed with diabetes, he or she is given a full medical examination. Their diabetes team will then work with them to make a programme of care which suits them and includes diabetes management goals — this may take the form of a record for them to keep. If they are lucky, they will also be seen by a diabetes specialist nurse. Insulin dependent diabetics are shown how to inject, look after their insulin and syringes and dispose of needles. They are also shown how to test their blood glucose and test for ketones, know what the results mean and what to do about them, and informed about hypoglycaemic episodes (hypos): when and why they may happen and how to deal with them. People on tablets are given instruction on blood or urine testing and have explained what the results mean and what to do about them.

People with Type 1 diabetes and tablet-controlled Type 2 diabetes are entitled to free prescriptions for medication, and free eye tests. Equipment such as blood glucose meters and finger pricking devices normally have to be purchased, but test strips, lancets, most insulin pens and pen needles are available on prescription. A prescription exemption certificate is necessary to obtain free prescriptions. People with diabetes also get free foot examinations and must be careful of getting infections in the feet. The nails on hands and feet often have brown marks on them which is a sure sign of diabetes.

Type 1
Insulin

Type 1 has been managed conventionally with insulin and a carbohydrate-based, low-fat diet. The carbohydrates in such a diet inevitably put large amounts of glucose in the bloodstream, and frequent insulin injections have to be administered to bring these high levels of glucose in the blood down to normal. When the illness is first diagnosed, most Type 1 diabetics are still producing some insulin, but this tapers off over time. Some researchers believe that if the illness is caught soon enough, a very high fat and low carbohydrate diet might obviate the need to inject insulin at all, or at least to need as much insulin. As it is, sufferers of Type 1 diabetes require insulin injections for the remainder of their lives. Unfortunately, insulin cannot be taken in tablet form because it would be broken down in the stomach before it could work. There are different types of insulin, and these can act very differently in different people. The insulin may be packaged in vials, cartridges or prefilled pens. The cartridges are used with pen injectors and the vials are used with syringes. Prefilled pens are disposable pen injectors, prefilled with insulin.

There are three main types of insulin, which are also available in various combinations in pre-mixed form. Rapid-acting analogue insulin can be injected just before or just after eating and lasts for between two and five hours. Long-acting analogue insulin is more slowly absorbed and lasts around 24 hours. It is taken only once a day, in the evening. Short-acting soluble insulin is usually taken 15 to 30 minutes before a meal and has its peak action within two to six hours after injecting. It can last for up to eight hours. Medium and long-acting usually have their peak activity between four and 12 hours after injecting and can last from eight to 30 hours. They are often used in combination with short-acting insulin.

A few years ago 'human' insulin replaced insulin derived from pigs. This new insulin was achieved using recombinant DNA technology, which means that it is genetically modified. It is not human at all, but a synthetic insulin chemically similar to human insulin. Many of the people I interviewed for this book complained of difficulty in controlling their blood sugar on the human insulin. It was first introduced, under pressure from the large drug companies, because many scientists and doctors believed that it would have many benefits over the older type of insulin precisely because it was 'human', but thousands of people complained to Diabetes UK that it made blood glucose levels harder to manage. Nevertheless, pig insulin is rarely used now, if at all.

LAURA

Laura, who is in her early thirties, has had diabetes since she was two years old, so she has known nothing else. She remembers that when she was a child her parents had to weigh all her food and work out the grams of carbohydrate it contained, and that she was not allowed to eat sugar. She sees a nutritionist regularly, and about three years ago gave up dairy and wheat. Her blood glucose levels have come down considerably since she made these changes to her diet, and so she needs less insulin at each injection than she used to. Where she used to use 20 units a day, now she only uses 12 units. She now uses an insulin pen four times a day, five minutes before eating, with the longer-acting Insulatard at bedtime to take her through the night. She was moved from porcine insulin to human insulin about eight years ago, but, in common with many other people I interviewed, finds the human insulin provides less control over blood glucose than the porcine insulin.

When I asked Laura how diabetes affected her life, she replied that diabetes is boring. She thinks about carbohydrates in general, without being particularly aware of the Glycaemic Index. Carbohydrates for her are usually rice, noodles, potatoes and rye bread. She does occasionally suffer from mood swings, and becomes irritated if her blood glucose levels are low. She has occasionally had hypos for no reason that she could identify, and actually passed out a couple of times.

Type 2

Type 2 diabetes is managed either with drugs or with diet and exercise alone. Occasionally people with Type 2 need insulin, either on its own or with drugs. I was surprised to find that several of the older Type 2 people I spoke to were on insulin.

GAY

Gay, a diabetes educator and nurse, has herself had Type 2 diabetes for 15 years. Three months ago she was put onto two different types of insulin: Lantus, which she takes at night, and Novo Rapid, a relatively new and extremely fast-acting insulin, immediately before a meal. She finds that the big advantage of Novo Rapid is that it is out of the system again within 3-5 hours, so reducing the risk of hypos and the necessity to have meals exactly on time. Unlike David, she has found the Lantus very effective, in that it does not have a significant peak and does last 24 hours, although it has the slight disadvantage of having to be taken at exactly the same time each night. Gay comments that this regime has completely revolutionised her life, in that she can now eat when she pleases. With her extensive knowledge of diabetes and how to manage it, she has always kept her blood glucose well under control, and her HbA1C has been consistent at 6.5% since she commenced insulin. However, she was delighted to find that, after three months on the new regime, it actually went down to 6.3%. Gay comments that with the Lantus and Novo Rapid regime, snacking should not really be necessary on a regular basis, as this regime mimics the body's own mechanism much more closely, i.e. a constant background low-level supply of insulin with post-prandial surges (that is, the Novo Rapid provides a surge of insulin to cope with the normal surge in blood glucose as a result of eating carbohydrates).

Drugs

Diabetes drugs work by lowering the blood glucose. They do this either by stimulating the pancreas to produce more insulin, or by helping the body to use the insulin that it does produce more effectively.

Sulphonylureas (e.g. Chlorpropamide) work by stimulating the cells in the pancreas to make more insulin. Unfortunately, they can cause your blood glucose levels to fall too low, causing hypoglycaemia, and can also cause weight gain. Prandial glucose regulators are shorter-acting. They are taken during a meal and work by stimulating your pancreas to produce more insulin. Biguanides (e.g. Metformin 'Glucophage') work in two ways. They help to stop the liver producing new glucose and also overcome insulin resistance by making insulin carry glucose into muscle and fat cells more effectively. Side effects include upset stomach, nausea and diarrhoea, and in some cases a serious condition called lactic acidosis. Alpha glucosidase inhibitors (e.g. Acarbose) work by slowing down the absorption of starchy foods from the intestine, thereby slowing down the rise in blood glucose after meals. Side effects can include wind, a feeling of fullness or diarrhoea. Thiazolidinediones (eg Pioglitazone) are a new family of tablets which overcome insulin resistance, enabling the body to use its own natural insulin more effectively. Side effects can include headaches, oedema (fluid retention), weight gain and, less commonly, upper respiratory tract infections. Finally, Guar Gum, which is a foodstuff rather than a drug, can reduce blood glucose levels if taken in adequate quantities, probably by slowing down the absorption of carbohydrates. It must be accompanied by large quantities of water, however, to prevent constipation, and it can cause flatulence.

JEAN

Jean was diagnosed with diabetes fourteen years ago when she had to go into hospital for a hip replacement. Two years before that she had visited her doctor complaining of excessive thirst, but at that time the doctor told her this was healthy and normal. She was prescribed Metformin to begin with, but this caused unpleasant gastric side-effects, so the dose was lowered and combined with insulin. Jean continued on this therapy until early 2003, but she is now on insulin alone as her pancreas is no longer able to make any insulin of its own. She takes 34 units of insulin a day, of two different types: one before breakfast which takes half an hour to kick in, and one at bedtime which works instantly. Jean has invested in a sophisticated battery-driven glucose meter called Medisense, which she uses on her arm rather than on her finger. She has found that different meters record different levels of blood glucose, which can be quite confusing.

When Jean feels she is about to have a hypo, she has learnt to take three glucose tablets all at once, and this brings her blood glucose up quickly enough to avert the hypo. If she wakes up with a low blood glucose reading of 5, she allows herself a spoonful of sugar in her tea, and this is enough to keep her blood sugar steady until breakfast. She breakfasts on half a grapefruit, one Weetabix with milk and an apple juice. This keeps her going through the morning and she finds she doesn't need a snack at all in the morning, though she may have a biscuit with tea in the afternoon. She makes lots of home-made soups, and eats plenty of fresh green vegetables. She normally eats fresh fruit for dessert, especially strawberries, but if she is out at a restaurant she might just try a spoonful of something like a cooked pudding. Jean seems to be very in tune with her diabetes, and knows only too well that if she eats sugar, sugar products, potatoes and bread her blood sugar will go sky-high, and this gives her the self-discipline to avoid or severely limit those foods. As she says, 'once you know you have diabetes, you know you've got to take care of it. If you don't, you're in trouble'.

Blood glucose monitoring (Type 1 and Type 2)

Blood glucose monitoring is an essential tool for controlling diabetes. It can help to maintain day-to-day control, detect hypoglycaemia, assess control during any illness, and help to provide information that can be used in the prevention of long-term complications. Blood glucose is monitored with the help of a blood glucose meter. There are many different sorts of glucose meter, some of which are downloadable to a computer so that you can keep track of your blood glucose fluctuations easily. Glucose meters measure blood glucose in mmol/L. The range of values the meter registers can be as wide as 0.6-33.3 mmol/L, whereas normal blood glucose is generally 3.5-8 mmol/L. Any values outside the normal range are registered as low or high.

HbA1C

This is a vital long-term blood sugar reading. The HbA1C score represents the level of glycosylation of haemoglobin in the blood (see page 17). The amount of haemoglobin which forms HbA1C will depend on the concentration of glucose that the haemoglobin is exposed to and the length of time it is exposed to a given concentration of glucose. So consistently high blood sugar over an extended period of time will cause a greater percentage of haemoglobin to be damaged in this way. A patient's HbA1C level is used to predict the likelihood of complications from diabetes. It is important to achieve a score of less than 7% on the HbA1C test. The HbA1C level changes slowly, over 10 weeks, unlike the blood sugar level which changes minute by minute, so it can be used as a 'quality control' test. Patients with diabetes who do not keep their HbA1C under 7% are at risk of developing serious long-term health problems including stroke, heart disease, diabetic retinopathy, blindness, kidney failure and amputation.

NUTRITIONAL MANAGEMENT OF DIABETES

People with diabetes have been bombarded with nutritional advice for many years. At the beginning of the twentieth century, they were advised to limit all food – not a very happy state of affairs. Later, in the 1920s, they were advised to eat high-fat diets on the basis that fat does not break down to glucose in the blood. In the 1970s and 1980s, the emphasis was on the amount of carbohydrate eaten, regardless of the type, and people with diabetes were advised to eat a set amount of carbohydrate at each meal. Nowadays the differences between types of carbohydrates are more clearly understood, and it is therefore much easier for a diabetic to control their blood glucose through diet, using the Glycaemic Index and Glycaemic Load.

The Glycaemic Index

It used to be thought that carbohydrates were either fast-release or slow-release, that is refined foods such as sugar were thought to release their sugar content rapidly, resulting in a rapid rise in blood glucose, while complex carbohydrates, such as whole grains, would release it more slowly. During the 1980's scientists conducted a series of trials in which volunteers fasted for some hours, then were given a single food to eat. The rise in their blood sugar was then measured over four hours to see the effect of each food on blood glucose. The researchers had two surprises. The first was that all carbohydrates, regardless of quality, cause a peak in blood glucose approximately 30 minutes after being eaten. The second was that some foods cause a much more dramatic rise than others. It was further discovered that some foods cause a higher blood glucose spike if they are cooked than if they are eaten raw, for example carrots.

Glucose was given a value of 100, and all other carbohydrates were ranked according to their effect on blood glucose levels. This ranking is known as the Glycaemic Index (GI). Carbohydrates that cause a sharp rise in blood glucose have the highest GI, whereas carbohydrates that have a gentler effect on blood glucose have a low GI. Various factors influence the GI value of a food: for example the gelatinisation of starch in pasta. If pasta is cooked until it is soft, the starch has had more time to absorb water, and consequently is more gelatinous than if the pasta is cooked 'al dente'. So the well-cooked pasta will have a higher GI than 'al dente' pasta. Similarly, if a food consists of small particles, for example white flour, it is easier for water and digestive enzymes to penetrate the particles, and consequently they will hit the bloodstream sooner than the large particles in stone-ground flour. So they will have a higher GI. Finally, and perhaps surprisingly, sugar is digested less rapidly than starch and thus has a relatively low GI (60-65). This is because sugar is not pure glucose, but consists of two molecules, one of glucose and one of fructose. Fructose produces a low blood sugar response, thus mitigating the effect of the glucose in sugar.

A low GI means a smaller rise in blood glucose levels after meals. A diet featuring low GI foods can help people lose weight and improve their sensitivity to insulin. Low GI foods can help re-fuel carbohydrate stores after exercise, improve diabetes control, keep you feeling fuller for longer and can prolong physical endurance.

RONA

Rona is a recently qualified nutritional therapist, and came to her new career largely because of her diabetes which made her interested in the whole topic of blood glucose and how to control it. She comes from a medical background, so when at the age of 22 she began to lose weight and grow very thin, while at the same time suffering from extreme thirst, she readily diagnosed herself as being diabetic. The condition progressed over a period of six weeks or so, during which she was climbing mountains in Scotland, so as she says, her energy appeared not be unduly affected at that time. She is still puzzled as to why she got diabetes – there was no particular stress in her life that she could think of, except the usual stresses a student might undergo, perhaps exacerbated in her case by a year in France where she had to write a thesis and make presentations in French. There is no diabetes in her family.

When she was finally diagnosed, Rona went into shock and denial about her diabetes. At that time she was using a syringe, but she refused to test her blood, hoping perhaps that the diabetes would go away if she ignored it. She was helped to accept it by her boss whose son was a diabetic and used an insulin pen. Rona, too, now uses an 'Act Rapid' pen, four times a day, with Insulatard at night.

Being nutritionally aware, Rona has learnt to manage her diabetes successfully using low GI foods. She finds lentils and porridge with raisins particularly helpful, and also relies on brown basmati rice and Warburtons multi-seed bread. Interestingly, in spite of their supposedly high GI rating, baked potatoes are still on Rona's menu, and they don't appear to raise her blood sugar unduly. She even eats ice cream sometimes – having discovered the Glycaemic Index in the last two years, she was delighted to find that ice cream did not score too highly. She mentioned the GI to her dietician, who was aware of it, but only had a casual acquaintance with it. Generally, Rona has not been impressed with dieticians and feels they could give more comprehensive and informed advice to people with diabetes. She has, however, had two successful pregnancies since becoming diabetic, and cannot praise more highly the care and monitoring she received while pregnant.

Rona is aware of when she's getting a hypo, and uses glucose sweets to bring her blood glucose level up quickly if necessary. As she says, 'the bottom line is: if you eat more than you inject, your blood sugar will not be controlled.'

The Glycaemic Load

The Glycaemic Load takes the concept of GI a step further, in providing a measure of total glycaemic response to a food or to a meal. The GL is equivalent to the GI value of a food multiplied by the amount of carbohydrate per serving and divided by 100. One unit of GL is equivalent to the glycaemic effect of 1g of pure glucose.

A food with a GL of 20 or more is high, a GL of 11 to 19 inclusive is medium, and a GL of 10 or less is low. Foods that have a low GI invariably have a low GL, while foods with an intermediate or high GI range from very low to very high GL. Therefore, you can reduce the GL of your diet by limiting foods that have both a high GI and a high carbohydrate content. A further complication is that acidic foods like lemon juice and vinegar lower the total glycaemic load, and fats such as olive oil slow the absorption of carbohydrates.

A meal contains a variety of different foods, so how do you work out the GI or GL value of a whole meal? Briefly, this is done by adding up all the grams of carbohydrate in the meal, working out what percentage each food contributes to the total carbohydrate content, and then multiplying this percentage by the GI value. An exact calculation is difficult and at times impossible, because the GI and GL of all foods have not yet been measured. I have therefore given an approximate guide for each recipe, stating whether a recipe is high, medium or low. The lists at the back of this book give both GI and GL values for reference. I have used the latest tables available, those published in the *American Journal of Clinical Nutrition* in 2002[15]. However, I would add the caveat that these are approximate only, and that the actual GI value may well be slightly different.

The Glycaemic Index and Glycaemic Load were never intended to be used in isolation. A food can have a low GI but still be high in saturated fat or have other undesirable qualities. So the recipes in this book have been chosen not only because they have low GI but also because they are healthy and well balanced.

What Proportion of Carbohydrates?

All food is made up of three macronutrients – protein, fat and carbohydrate. Because diabetes is a disorder of carbohydrate metabolism, a person with diabetes needs to know what proportion of carbohydrates in the diet will enable them to control their blood sugar most effectively.

The standard advice given by both the American Diabetes Association and Diabetes UK is still to follow a high carbohydrate, low fat diet, even though research is favouring a more balanced ratio. The ratio usually recommended is 15% protein, 55% carbohydrate and 30% fat. However, it doesn't seem logical to base the diet on carbohydrates, as these are the foods that people with diabetes, by definition, have the most difficulty metabolising. A high intake of carbohydrates, particularly of high GI carbohydrates, leads to consistently high blood glucose levels. The solution would appear to be a lower carbohydrate diet, replacing carbohydrates not with saturated fat, but with modest amounts of essential fats and more protein. This approach is supported by a recent preliminary study in which people with Type 2 diabetes achieved lower blood glucose and lower blood fats following a lower carbohydrate, higher protein diet (30% protein, 40% carbohydrate and 30% fat) than those on the standard 15:55:30 diet mentioned above[16]. The lower carbohydrate, higher protein diet is known by researchers as the 'prudent' dietary pattern. It is characterised by a high intake of vegetables, pulses, fruit and whole grains, and a low intake of red meat, processed meat, high-fat dairy products and refined grains. It is not the same as the Atkins diet, which contains far less carbohydrate, more protein and typically a high intake of saturated fat too. The 'prudent' diet is the pattern on which I have based the recipes in this book, although in practice it is quite difficult to achieve that level of protein over the course of a day's menus, particularly if you are avoiding or limiting red meat which is the richest source of dietary protein.

Vegetables

It is important to eat a wide variety of vegetables. They are rich in fibre and nutrients and help to protect the cardiovascular system and nerves from glycosylation. Avoid cooked starchy root vegetables especially potatoes and parsnips as they have a very high

GI value. **Beetroot** should be eaten raw, as it contains chromium, as do the beet greens. **Mushrooms** also contain chromium. Certain vegetables are particularly beneficial, such as **onions** and **garlic**, as they are able to reduce blood sugar. They contain active ingredients that appear to increase insulin in the blood by preventing it being inactivated by the liver.[17] **Jerusalem artichokes, broccoli, celery, cabbage, chicory, Chinese cabbage, courgettes, kale, radishes** and **tomatoes** are also among the recommended 'nutriceuticals' for diabetes[18]. **Avocados** and **olives** are particularly high in monounsaturated fatty acids, and are good choices. Finally, mung beans, usually eaten as **beansprouts**, are thought to be beneficial as an antidiabetic, low glycaemic index food, rich in antioxidants[19]. Antioxidants have been found to be very important in relation to the development of Type 2 diabetes, particularly vitamin E. In a recent study, researchers found that the highest long term vitamin E intake was significantly associated with a reduced risk of Type 2 diabetes, compared to subjects with the lowest intake. Good sources of vitamin E include spinach, eggs, meat, poultry, fish, nuts and seeds, avocado and tomatoes. Those with the highest intakes of a carotenoid found in sweet peppers, sweetcorn and watermelon also had a 40% reduced risk of Type 2 diabetes.[20]

Fruit

Choose low GI fruits such as **apples** and **pears** and avoid high GI fruits such as melon and bananas. **Grapefruit**, which has a very low GI, may be one of the healthiest dietary choices for people with diabetes and for those trying to lose weight, because it contains enzymes that help control insulin spikes that occur after a meal, thus freeing the digestive system to process food more efficiently, with the result that fewer nutrients are stored as fat.

Consumption of fruit should, however, be moderate. One rather startling finding of interest to people with diabetes is that apparently fruit is getting sweeter. Recent American government research found that apples can now comprise up to 15% sugar compared with 8%-10% three decades ago. Similar increases have been reported in pineapples, pears and bananas. It appears that farming techniques have changed to meet consumer demand. For example, in apples this is partly due to new varieties and partly to how they are picked and stored so that they retain more sugar. Most fruit juice provides about 10 grams of sugar per 100 grams – about the same as a cola drink. It is wise to avoid fruit juice for this reason, or to dilute it with water. Vegetable juices are a better choice, and you will find several delicious recipes for vegetable juices in the drinks section.

Protein foods

Amino acids, the breakdown products of protein foods, are normally considered as the 'building blocks' of the body, in that their primary role is that of maintenance and repair. But our bodies will also make glucose from protein. Since glucose, usually sourced from carbohydrates, is what gives us energy, it is important for a person with diabetes who is limiting their carbohydrates to eat enough protein. Protein also has the effect of slowing the absorption of glucose from carbohydrates, so always make sure you eat a small portion of protein at each snack or meal. Choose fish, especially the oily fish such as organic or wild **salmon** and **mackerel, live natural yoghurt, cottage cheese, pulses, quinoa, soya** and **poultry**, as these are low in saturated fats.

It may be wise to limit the amount of red meat you eat if you have diabetes. A study has indicated that the consumption of red meat, which contains haem iron, is associated with an increased risk of Type 2 diabetes[21]. The findings also revealed that people with haemochromatosis, a disease in which the body takes in too much iron with food, are more likely to develop diabetes. This may be because iron is a catalyst in the formation of dangerous free radicals.

Whole grains

Although carbohydrates should be limited, they should definitely not be avoided completely. But it is important to choose the right sort of carbohydrates – vegetables, fruit, pulses, and whole grains. Studies have shown that those with the highest intake of whole grains and cereal fibre are less likely to develop metabolic syndrome, which predisposes to diabetes.

One of the most beneficial grains for people with diabetes is **buckwheat,** which is readily available in health food shops. It is not related to wheat, and is not even, technically, a grain, but a fruit. Several studies have shown than buckwheat may help increase insulin sensitivity. Previous studies have shown how a component of buckwheat called chiro-inositol may prompt cells to become more receptive to insulin. Chiro-inositol is relatively high in buckwheat and rarely found in other foods. Of all the seeds analysed, only mung beans have more. Some diabetics don't see any change in blood glucose levels when they consume buckwheat, but it is possible that the compound is still helping their bodies to use glucose more effectively. Also, there are a couple of small studies published in China and India indicating that people with Type 2 diabetes who consumed buckwheat had better glycaemic control. The glycaemic index of buckwheat has been extensively tested and is about 54, and its glycaemic load is 16, which is medium.

In the recipes I have used **buckwheat, pearl barley, quinoa,**

brown rice, polenta, whole wheat and **amaranth,** as these all have a low GI value. Whole grains contain chromium, needed for carbohydrate metabolism, and lots of minerals and vitamins. Avoid any products made with refined white flour. Not only is it high GI, but it is almost devoid of nutritional value.

The gluten grains (barley, rye, oats and wheat) can pose potential problems for people with diabetes, and a small proportion (about 5%) of Type 1 diabetics are coeliac, which means they cannot digest these grains at all. I have therefore included some gluten-free recipes. However, many people intolerant to wheat but not actually coeliac can tolerate oats and barley, though they do contain some gluten.

I have only included one bread recipe, and that is for barley bread, because barley has a relatively low GI. The fibre content of barley accounts for its ability to lower cholesterol and glucose, and the beta-glucans it contains may also reduce appetite by slowing down emptying of the stomach and stabilising blood sugar. Bread should not really be used as a staple by people with diabetes owing to its high carbohydrate content. If you cannot do without bread, it might be worth searching out Burgen Soy Lin bread as it is the lowest GI bread ever tested (see Useful Addresses).

Dairy products

It appears that dairy products cause an unusual increase in insulin secretion. This may be because cow's milk proteins are designed to stimulate growth in young calves, whose normal growth rate consists of doubling their birth weight within the first month. Insulin does more than drive glucose into the cells – it also encourages the uptake of essential fatty acids and proteins, needed for growth. I therefore do not use cow's milk in the recipes, but substitute **soya milk** or **rice milk.** Butter is acceptable in small amounts as it is nearly all fat and contains virtually no protein. I do use butter in baking and in recipes where the taste of the fat is important, and I also use a little Parmesan and goats cheese for flavour where nothing else can substitute. Live yoghurt and a little cottage cheese are also acceptable.

Fats and oils

Fat does not increase blood glucose levels, but that does not mean that fats can be eaten indiscriminately, for there are good fats and bad fats. It is very important to avoid scrupulously any trans-fatty acids or hydrogenated fats (most cooking fats, margarines and processed foods) and refined oils. A large, long-term study of 84,000 women recently found that trans-fatty acids can raise a woman's risk of Type 2 diabetes, while substituting foods rich in trans fats with those that contain polyunsaturated fats could reduce the risk by about 40%[22].

The monounsaturated fats, such as **extra virgin olive oil**, and the omega-3 fatty acids found in oily fish and nuts, actually lower serum triglycerides and contribute to glycaemic control in people with diabetes. Population studies on the peoples of Greenland have suggested that fish oil might help protect against diabetes. These people, who live on whale blubber, are often overweight and could be expected to have diabetes and heart disease, but they do not. Researchers think this is because of the high proportion of omega-3 fatty acids in their diet.

There are only three fats and oils that should be used for cooking – extra virgin olive oil, virgin coconut oil and organic butter. For salad dressings, extra virgin olive oil or any of the delicious cold-pressed seed or nut oils may be used, such as walnut oil and flax seed oil (rich in omega-3 fatty acids), avocado oil or pumpkin seed oil. For spreading, try almond or hazelnut butter or tahini (sesame seed paste). Organic butter is also an acceptable choice, as it is a rich source of easily absorbed vitamin A and all the other fat-soluble vitamins (E, K, and D). It is rich in trace minerals, especially selenium, a powerful antioxidant. It has appreciable amounts of butyric acid, used by the colon as an energy source, and lauric acid, a medium-length long-chain fatty acid (MCFA).

Coconut oil has some interesting properties that make it very suitable for people with diabetes. It helps to regulate blood sugar, and it also raises the metabolic rate, causing the body to burn up more calories and thus promoting weight loss. A faster metabolic rate stimulates increased production of insulin and increases absorption of glucose into cells, thus helping both Type 1 and Type 2 diabetics.[23] Coconut oil is composed of about 50% lauric acid. Like other MCFAs, lauric acid is digested and processed differently from other fats. It is sent directly to the liver where it is immediately converted into energy – just like a carbohydrate. Numerous studies have shown that replacing long chain fatty acids with MCFA results in a decrease in body weight gain and a reduction in fat deposition[24]. Furthermore, reports from India reveal that Type 2 diabetes there has increased as people have abandoned coconut oil in favour of refined vegetable oils.[25] Organic coconut oil is available from Higher Nature (see Useful Addresses).

Acid and Fermented Foods
The acetic acid in vinegar and the citric acid in lemon and lime juice are able to actually reduce blood glucose levels by slowing the speed at which the stomach empties into the intestine[26]. In one

study the glucose response with vinegar was 31% lower than without it. In another study vinegar significantly reduced the glycaemic index of a starchy meal from 100 to 64[27]. Fermented foods such as pickles and sauerkraut may have the same effect.

Nuts and Seeds

Nuts and seeds are nutrient-dense and contain essential fats, protein and some fibre. The best nuts are those with a higher proportion of monounsaturated fatty acids, such as **macadamia nuts, hazelnuts, pecans** and **almonds**. Almonds are particularly important for people with diabetes or metabolic syndrome. A recent study found that a low calorie diet supplemented with almonds not only helped people to lose weight but also enabled Type 1 diabetics to reduce their medication.[28] Nuts and seeds are rich in magnesium. Findings from a recent large long-term study suggest a significant inverse association between magnesium intake and diabetes risk. Furthermore, diabetics are usually deficient in magnesium[29]. It is therefore important to increase consumption of major food sources of magnesium, such as whole grains, nuts, seeds and green leafy vegetables.

Nuts and seeds can be eaten as a snack with a piece of fruit, or ground and added to porridge, live yoghurt or vegetable juices to increase fibre intake. Avoid salted or dry roasted nuts.

Sugar and sweeteners

Sugar consumption and the incidence of diabetes appear to have kept pace with each other in the developing world. However, there is no proof that sugar consumption is the direct cause of diabetes. Indeed, the story is much more complex. It's not sugar that causes diabetes, but rather a combination of genetic and environmental factors, some of which I have outlined earlier. But even if sugar doesn't cause diabetes, should people who have the disease avoid it? In fact, the American Diabetes Association (ADA) stopped recommending that people with diabetes avoid sugar in May 1994. Similarly, Diabetes UK no longer forbids sugar. However, there are plenty of reasons why diabetics, along with everyone else, should avoid refined sugar at all costs. Reducing the amount of sugar in the diet helps to reduce weight which in turn improves glycaemic control[30].

White sugar is particularly damaging as the B vitamins and trace minerals such as zinc, manganese, chromium, selenium and cobalt are all removed by the refining process. As these substances are necessary for the body to metabolise sugar, the sugar squanders these nutrients from the body's reserves. Sugar also suppresses the immune system and has a hand in numerous other conditions, such as elevated cholesterol, kidney damage, depression, hormonal imbalance, free radical formation, hypertension, migraines and osteoporosis.

Unfortunately many doctors and dieticians are still advising people with diabetes to replace sugar with substances that could be even more harmful in the long run – sweeteners. There are five intense (artificial) sweeteners that are permitted for use in the UK: aspartame, saccharin, acesulfame potassium (acesulfame K), cyclamate and sucralose. These sweeteners have their own disadvantages, and should be avoided because they promote a sweet tooth, increase cravings for sweet foods and make it more difficult to lose weight. A possible explanation is that when you eat an artificial sweetener, the body prepares itself to digest carbohydrates which then fail to materialise. When you do subsequently eat some carbohydrate the body compromises by creating a greater than normal rise in blood sugar. Not only that, but some sweeteners have more sinister drawbacks. Aspartame is a neurotoxin[31]. It is processed using methanol which is highly toxic. Complaints about its effects range from headaches to seizures. Sucralose, which is marketed as Splenda, has no calories and is about 600 times sweeter than sugar. It is produced by chlorinating sugar, which involves chemically changing the structure of the sugar molecules. Sucralose has not been much tested on humans, but one small study of diabetic patients using sucralose showed a statistically significant increase in the long-term blood glucose marker, HbA1C.

Fructose is the form of sugar found in fruit, as its name suggests. When naturally contained within a whole food, it causes no problems. However, it is commercially extracted and refined from corn, and is often found in processed foods as high fructose corn syrup. It does not affect the blood glucose as much as sucrose, but it is thought to lead to the formation of advanced glycation end products (AGEs), which have been implicated in many degenerative diseases such as cataracts. Animal studies have found that fructose consumption contributes to insulin resistance, an impaired tolerance to glucose, high blood pressure, and elevated levels of triglycerides. Although the data in humans is not quite as conclusive as the animal trials, the researchers report that an increased intake of fructose may increase body weight and encourage insulin resistance, both of which are risk factors for Type 2 diabetes. Finally, evidence is mounting that many people who experience irritable bowel syndrome and other gastrointestinal discomfort may be suffering from fructose intolerance.

There are two forms of sweetener that are safer than aspartame and sucralose. The first is **FOS** (Fructo-oligosaccharides), obtainable from health food shops. FOS can be used in baking and to sweeten stewed fruit. It is mildly sweet and nourishes the beneficial bacteria in the gut. However, it can cause flatulence and bloating. The second is **Stevia,** a member of the chrysanthemum family. This natural sweetener, which comes from Paraguay, has been used for centuries, and is used today in South America, South East Asia and the Far East. However, it is banned in the EU and the USA as a foodstuff. The EC Scientific Committee on Food (SCF) came to the conclusion that it has the potential to produce adverse effects in the male reproductive system that could affect fertility, and that it could damage DNA. It is therefore highly controversial. Many diabetics do use it, and in recent studies it has proved to have beneficial effects on Type 2 diabetes and high blood pressure[32].

I think the best approach to sugar and sweeteners is to try to re-educate one's palate, so that one does not crave sweet foods. This is possible, although it takes time. You may be helped by using a supplement containing magnesium, chromium or glutamine (see pages 38-39). Fresh fruit can fulfil the need for sweetness without the health concerns attached to artificial sweeteners or stevia.

Drinks
Tea, coffee, cola drinks and chocolate
All these drinks contain stimulants such as caffeine which produce spikes in blood glucose levels. Preliminary findings from a small study suggest that drinking moderate amounts of coffee may decrease insulin sensitivity in healthy people by as much as 15%[33]. The finding may have serious health implications, especially with regard to people who already have Type 2 diabetes, because this effect is the reverse of that of prescription diabetes drugs such as metformin (Glucophage), so that if you take a drug for Type 2 diabetes and wash it down with coffee, you may be cancelling out the effects of the drug

On the other side of the argument, however, a recent large-scale study revealed that regular daily coffee drinking may *reduce* the risk of developing Type 2 diabetes. Though caffeine appears to be the primary source of benefits, the study's authors suggested that the potassium, magnesium, and antioxidants in coffee might improve the body's response to insulin. The study had limitations, however. The researchers could not be certain that coffee decreases the incidence of Type 2 diabetes, as it could be something else about coffee drinkers that protects them from diabetes.[34] Other studies, from Sweden and Holland, have shown that regular coffee consumption may protect against the development of Type 2 diabetes.[35, 36] However, coffee has other disadvantages, as it may interfere with your body's ability to keep homocysteine and cholesterol levels in check, probably by inhibiting the action of the vitamins folate, B12 or B6, and it is associated with increased risk of stroke and rheumatoid arthritis. Studies have also shown that the caffeine in coffee can raise blood pressure. It also raises the levels of adrenaline by up to 500%, which may be connected to its ability to decrease insulin sensitivity. Since coffee is a stimulant it will only worsen any symptoms of insomnia and anxiety and should definitely be avoided.

Fizzy drinks and cordials should be avoided as they are high in sugar. Diet drinks contain sweeteners such as aspartame and should also be avoided. This also applies to the currently fashionable flavoured waters. Instead, drink **herbal teas, water, dandelion coffee, green** or **jasmine tea, hot water** with **lemon** or **ginger**.

Avoid fruit juice – fruit juice is a concentrated form of carbohydrate – the sugars in fruit juice contribute to major distortions of insulin balance.

Alcohol

It appears that moderate alcohol consumption, as opposed to total abstinence, is associated with a decreased incidence of heart disease in people with diabetes, according to a recent review of the scientific literature on the subject.[37] A French study has found that insulin resistance is minimal in individuals with regular mild to moderate alcohol consumption and increases in both heavy drinkers and subjects without any alcohol consumption at all[38]. Moderate alcohol consumption is usually taken to mean not more than two or three units of alcohol per day. However, some people should not consume alcohol because of the medication they take for diabetes or other conditions.

The dangers of heavy drinking are even more acute for people with diabetes than for anyone else. The risks of heavy or continuous alcohol intake include hypoglycaemia, glucose intolerance, and ketone and lactate accumulation.[39] The growing alcohol consumption in young people, particularly in young women, may be a risk factor for the development of Type 2 diabetes. A recently completed 10 year study examining the relationship between alcohol consumption and the incidence of Type 2 diabetes in women found that, whereas light alcohol consumption may be associated with a lower risk, this benefit may not persist at higher levels[40].

Convenience foods

Convenience foods and ready meals should be avoided whenever possible. Read labels carefully to check for saturated fat, fibre and sugar content. Hidden sugars include corn syrup, dextrose and fructose. Low fat foods are by default high in carbohydrates and often in sugar too.

Salt

For years doctors have told people to restrict salt, even those who do not have high blood pressure. But a recent study from Columbia University Medical School shows that salt restriction raises blood sugar and insulin levels, while a diet high in salt loading apparently lowers them. The conclusion of the study was that a high sodium intake may improve glucose tolerance and insulin resistance, especially in diabetic subjects."[41] This was a small preliminary study and should itself be taken with a pinch of salt! I would advise very moderate use of salt, and to avoid highly salted foods. I usually use sea salt as it contains some trace minerals and is very concentrated so you need to use less of it.

Herbs and spices

Several culinary herbs have been shown to help improve the action of insulin in lowering blood sugar levels. These include coriander, bay, juniper berries, fenugreek seed, cloves, turmeric, and cinnamon, and you will find many uses for these spices in the recipes that follow.

Cinnamon is particularly effective. A recent study reported in *Diabetes Care* found that just 1g (less than half a teaspoon) of cinnamon per day reduced blood glucose levels by 20%, as well as triglycerides, LDL cholesterol, and total cholesterol in 60 people with Type 2 diabetes.[42] In the study, lower blood glucose levels were maintained for 20 days after stopping the cinnamon capsules. This may mean that it is not necessary to take cinnamon every day to produce benefit.

The active ingredient in cinnamon is a flavonoid called methylhydroxychalcone polymer (MHCP) which has insulin-like activity. It appears that MHCP works both in synergy with insulin and on its own to regulate glucose metabolism. It would be wise for any diabetic wishing to try cinnamon to work with their doctor or diabetes nurse to monitor progress.

Exercise caution if using large amounts of whole cinnamon. It has both fat-soluble and water-soluble fractions and there is some evidence that high levels of the fat-soluble fractions of cinnamon could be cause for concern if a person is taking 1g per day. One solution is to make an infusion of cinnamon by boiling it in water, then straining the liquid through muslin and discarding the pulp. The liquid, which will contain only the water-soluble fraction, can then be drunk as a tea or used in food.

Snacks

Snacks are very important to people with diabetes, though less so to those who are using a combination of a basal insulin such as Lantus together with a fast-acting insulin at mealtimes. For those who are less able to keep their blood sugar levels even, snacks should be consumed between meals. But they have to be balanced snacks. A snack consisting solely of carbohydrate will have a marked effect on blood glucose, whereas a combination of protein and a low GI carbohydrate will keep the blood glucose more even. An exception is when people with diabetes, usually Type 1, experience a hypoglycaemic episode (a hypo), when their blood glucose level dips below 70mg/dl and they feel shaky and weak, or perhaps start talking incoherently. Then they need a high GI carbohydrate snack, and they need it fast, or they are in danger of passing out. Most diabetics have their own personal choice of high glucose food to raise their blood sugar quickly. Some people use pure glucose tablets, whilst some use orange juice or sugar lumps.

NUTRITIONAL SUPPLEMENTATION

It is a good idea for people with diabetes to boost their diet with nutritional supplements, but this should be done with your doctor's full knowledge and in conjunction with a qualified nutritional therapist. If you are taking prescribed medication for diabetes, the medication may need adjustment if you start to take natural remedies. This is because some supplements could potentiate the action of the drugs you are taking, i.e. make them more powerful, so you may need less medication.

Multi-vitamin

It is advisable for people with diabetes to take a good quality multiple vitamin because of their increased risk of cardiovascular disease, nerve and kidney damage and blindness. A small-scale double blind study of older people with Type 2 diabetes has shown that people with diabetes can reduce the risk of infection by supplementing with a multi-vitamin.[43]

Vitamins C and E

One out of three people with diabetes develops kidney disease in their lifetime. But if the warning signs are noted before kidney function is actually reduced, treatment may prevent further damage. One of the most valuable markers of a diabetic's kidney health is urinary albumin excretion rate (AER). Albumin is a protein synthesised in the liver that works to transport various substances in the blood stream. A Danish study has shown that vitamin C (1250mg/day) and vitamin E (680iu/day) had kidney-protective effects on a group of diabetic subjects with high AER levels. The AER levels decreased significantly in the patients taking the vitamins.

A recent study showed that vitamin C appears to reduce levels of C-reactive protein (CRP) which is an indicator of inflammation. There is a growing body of evidence that chronic inflammation is linked to an increased risk of heart disease and diabetes[44]. Long-term adverse health effects occur when inflammation persists at low levels. This chronic inflammation, with persistent low levels of CRP, has been found among smokers and Type 2 diabetics, as well as among people who are overweight.

Vitamin D
Chronic inflammation and CRP levels, along with associated risk of diabetes and other inflammatory conditions, have been shown to be lowered with vitamin D supplementation.[45]

Vitamin D deficiency has been associated with insulin deficiency and insulin resistance.[46] It has also been hypothesised that vitamin D deficiency may be a major factor in the development of Type 1 diabetes in children[47]. The best dietary sources of Vitamin D are eggs and oily fish. But the best strategy is exposure to sunlight in the summer months which causes the body to manufacture vitamin D. Between October and March in the UK, cod liver oil as a vitamin D supplement of not more than 1,000iu per day may be advisable.

Alpha-lipoic acid
Alpha-lipoic acid (ALA) is a powerful antioxidant that can help lower blood sugar, decrease glucose and insulin levels, increase insulin sensitivity, decrease insulin resistance, inhibit glycosylation (HbA1C levels) and help promote and maintain eye health. It has also been shown in studies to alleviate diabetic neuropathy at doses of 600mg a day. It is used in Germany to treat diabetes.

In addition, ALA can create new molecules of vitamins C and E from their molecular building blocks. There is research showing that ALA lowers blood-sugar levels in normal, or non-diabetic, subjects as well as in those with diabetes.

Essential fatty acids
Fish oils contain two fatty acids – Eicosapentaenoic Acid (EPA), and Docosahexaenoic Acid (DHA). People with diabetes have been

shown to have markedly lower levels of DHA than other people[48]. In one study, three months of daily supplementation with DHA produced a "clinically significant" improvement in insulin sensitivity in overweight people[49]. This study used only DHA, but ideally EPA and DHA should always be taken in a balanced dose. The EPA and DHA probably work by improving the sensitivity of insulin receptors. Not only will this help diabetes, but it will also help control weight. In an encouraging new study, doctors in Denmark have concluded that fish oil supplementation can help Type 2 diabetics reduce the high levels of fat present in their blood. Study participants who took fish oil lowered their ratio of LDL to HDL by almost one percent. Those taking corn oil, which is largely omega 6, raised their ratio by four percent.[50]

Evening Primrose Oil (EPO) contains Gamma Linoleic Acid (GLA), one of whose functions is to protect the nerves. The body normally makes GLA from alpha-linoleic acid (ALA), but diabetes can reduce the body's ability to produce GLA, and therefore neuropathy, or nerve damage, is a common complication of diabetes. Neuropathy can occur in any part of the body, but in diabetics it is particularly prominent in the legs and feet, causing numbness, tingling, pain, skin ulcers, and other problems.

Diabetics given GLA supplements were proven in a Glasgow study to be totally protected from small blood vessel damage in the eyes and peripheries, due to improved blood flow. Evening primrose oil supplements reduce elevated total cholesterol levels found in many diabetics, and a recent review of 22 clinical studies of evening primrose oil showed that all but six of the studies confirmed EPO to have a positive effect in treating diabetic neuropathy.

Magnesium
Research suggests that supplementing with magnesium can help promote healthy insulin production. It can also reduce the craving for sweet foods that can contribute to the development of Type 2 diabetes[51]. Researchers have assessed six years of data on more than 12,000 people who participated in the Atherosclerosis Risk in Communities Study. The researchers found no significant correlation between low dietary intake of magnesium and diabetes risk. However, while that might seem at first like a paradox, body stores of magnesium can be depleted by a high intake of starches or alcohol, while diuretics and some prescription drugs can increase urinary excretion of magnesium. Menstruation and stress can also contribute to magnesium depletion. Other studies have shown a clear association between low serum magnesium levels and an elevated risk of type 2 diabetes. Now a new study has shown that

there may even be a correlation between magnesium depletion, Type 2 diabetes and Alzheimers disease (AD)[52]. Some researchers believe that high blood glucose levels may play a role in the abnormal processing of a protein that prompts the accumulation of destructive peptide tangles in the brain.

Coenzyme Q10
Coenzyme Q10 is a powerful antioxidant which may help to maintain a healthy heart. Those doctors who are inclined towards a more natural approach have been using it successfully for years to help diabetic and pre-diabetic patients improve their fasting blood glucose and fasting insulin levels[53]. 50 mg a day can be beneficial, but it is an expensive supplement.

Chromium
Chromium appears to be the most useful mineral in preventing Type 2 diabetes for a couple of reasons. It is one of the major components of glucose tolerance factor, a molecule that improves the ability of insulin to lower blood glucose levels. In fact, without adequate chromium, insulin cannot be activated and blood glucose goes out of control[54]. Chromium can also significantly reduce sugar cravings. A study in India found that chromium supplementation seemed to improve glycaemic control in Type 2 diabetic patients. This effect appeared to be due to an increase in insulin action rather than stimulation of insulin secretion.[55]

Chromium helps stabilise blood sugar levels and can be beneficial in Type 2 diabetes. It also helps to reduce heart disease due to its effect in improving insulin utilisation and decreasing insulin requirements. Precisely because it is effective, however, people with diabetes may have an increased risk of hypoglycaemic episodes (hypos) when taking chromium supplements as self-medication, so blood sugar levels should be strictly monitored while taking chromium. Chromium is found in brewer's yeast, liver, beef, beetroot, black pepper, thyme and mushrooms. It is also found in whole grains, but the refining process removes chromium as it does other minerals, so refined grains lack it.

B-Complex
The entire B-complex is important in blood sugar metabolism, but make sure that the supplement you choose contains at least 15 to 25 milligrams of niacin and 50 to 100 milligrams of niacinamide (both are forms of vitamin B3). Niacin is another crucial component of glucose tolerance factor. Niacinamide helps protect pancreatic islet cells against the ultimate exhaustion that can be created by years of insulin overproduction.

Vitamin B6 (pyridoxine)
Along with folic acid and B12, B6 has been found to help reduce the levels of homocysteine in the blood. Homocysteine is a toxic metabolite of protein digestion, high levels of which are associated with increased risk of heart disease. One study found that high homocysteine levels were associated with diabetic neuropathy[56]. Not only that, but people with diabetes are often deficient in vitamin B6.

Biotin
It is a good idea to take an additional biotin supplement, even though this nutrient is found in most multivitamins. In order for biotin to really help metabolise blood sugar once it gets into the cells, you should take 1 to 2 milligrams a day — multivitamins don't usually provide nearly enough. B-complex and biotin can help inhibit glycosylation of proteins in diabetics.

Vitamin K
Protecting the body from insulin resistance appears to be one of vitamin K's many roles in the body. Dark green leafy vegetables are excellent sources of vitamin K, so make sure to eat plenty of broccoli and cabbage. It is not usually necessary to supplement vitamin K.

Vanadium
Twenty years ago, researchers were finding that small doses of this trace mineral could significantly improve blood sugar regulation. A word of caution, however: as with many of the trace minerals, there is a very narrow line between the benefits and toxicity of vanadium. While it can be an effective addition to your diabetes prevention and treatment programme, more does not necessarily mean better. Vanadium does occur naturally in food, such as pepper, dill, radishes, eggs, buckwheat, and oats. As for supplementing with vanadium, the best plan is to find a multivitamin that contains vanadium as vanadyl sulphate.

Pycnogenol
In a recent study, researchers found that Type 2 diabetes patients had lower blood sugar and healthier blood vessels after supplementing with Pycnogenol, a French maritime pine tree bark extract. The researchers report that the patients were able to significantly lower their glucose levels when they supplemented with 50-200 mg of the supplement. Pycnogenol has also been shown to improve cardiovascular problems prevailing in diabetics. Studies have found that Pycnogenol reduces high blood pressure, platelet aggregation and LDL cholesterol and enhances circulation. [57]

HERBAL SUPPLEMENTS

- **Ginseng** is believed by the Chinese to stimulate the release of insulin from the pancreas and increase the number of insulin receptors. In one clinical trial quite low doses of Asian ginseng (Panax ginseng) had beneficial blood-sugar lowering effects on Type 2 diabetes.[58]
- **Bitter melon** (Momordica Charantia or karela), a fruit indigenous to South America and Asia, has a blood sugar lowering effect in diabetes and appears to increase the healthy regeneration of insulin-secreting beta cells in the pancreas.[59] Modern science has confirmed that the juice and unripe fruit of this plant have powerful blood sugar reducing effects, mainly due to two compounds it contains, one of which, momordica, is chemically similar to insulin.
- **Gymnema Sylvestre,** is a tropical forest plant from India, is known as 'gurmar' which means 'sugar-destroyer'. It stimulates the pancreas to produce insulin and reduces the craving for sweet foods. It is also reported to assist with beta cell regeneration. Clinical trials have found it to considerably reduce blood sugar in over 90% of patients.[60]
- **Garcinia cambogia** is a yellowish pumpkin-shaped tropical tree fruit native to India that contains hydroxycitric acid (HCA), which has been shown to suppress fatty acid synthesis and food intake, in addition to sparing the use of carbohydrate in the body while causing an increase in fat oxidation. However, these were animal studies, and so far human studies have not confirmed these findings.
- **Chinese herbs.** It is estimated that more than 200 species of plants exhibit hypoglycaemic properties, including many common plants, such as pumpkin, wheat, celery, wax guard and lotus root as well as bitter melon. To date, hundreds of herbs and traditional Chinese medicine formulae have been reported to have been used for the treatment of diabetes.[61]

A NOTE ABOUT GLUCOSAMINE

Recent animal studies as well as some anecdotal evidence have suggested that glucosamine might increase insulin resistance and therefore could be harmful to diabetics. It appears that glucosamine may raise blood glucose in about 50% of people with diabetes. So if you have Type 2 diabetes and want to take glucosamine and chondroitin to relieve your arthritis symptoms, be sure that the doctor is aware that you're taking it and closely monitors your glucose levels.

EXERCISE

The single most important factor in controlling (and preventing) insulin resistance and adult-onset diabetes mellitus is exercise. Regular exercise can lower insulin resistance and improve Type 2 diabetes. The Finnish Diabetes Prevention Study (2001) by Tuomilehto and colleagues demonstrated conclusively that life-style modification could thwart the development of diabetes. This 10-year study of 522 people with impaired glucose tolerance showed that their risk of developing diabetes was reduced by 80 per cent if they lost 10 kg. A second study showed that people who did some aerobic-type exercise that caused them to "sweat a little" for 30 minutes three times a week cut their risk of going from Metabolic Syndrome (see page 13) to diabetes by nearly 60%.

Exercise will decrease blood sugar if the exercise is prolonged and strenuous. Blood sugars should be monitored every 10 minutes when starting an exercise routine to check for hypoglycaemia (low blood sugar) and test if the exercise needs to be covered with carbohydrate to compensate for hypoglycaemia. Anaerobic exercise (i.e. weightlifting) is ideal for diabetics because it lowers blood sugar more than aerobic exercise (running, biking, swimming, etc.), and it causes insulin to be much more efficient in transporting glucose into the cells.

Perhaps more important, however, exercise improves insulin sensitivity (a major problem in diabetes). Older people hampered by arthritis generally don't exercise enough and often become sedentary. This lack of activity causes insulin resistance, obesity, elevated fasting blood sugar and even elevated cholesterol. One large 16-year longitudinal study of 5,000 men has found that physical activity causes a reduction in insulin resistance. In the study, the risk for Type 2 diabetes decreased progressively with increasing levels of physical activity. The authors maintain that insulin resistance definitely plays an important role in the development of diabetes[62].

All of the muscles need exercise in order to maximise glucose absorption. There is a difference between aerobic and anaerobic exercise. Anaerobic exercise is done in short sessions and improves muscle tone. Aerobic exercise is usually done in longer sessions and improves heart rate. When it comes to improving insulin sensitivity (reducing insulin resistance), most research supports aerobic activity. Earlier research indicated that only high-intensity aerobic activity reduced insulin resistance, but more recent research indicates that even low-intensity aerobic exercise, such as walking, helps. Only recently has anaerobic exercise been given equal billing with aerobic activity for controlling and managing diabetes.

When should you exercise? Since we expect blood glucose levels to rise after meals, then diabetics would do well to engage in physical activity after meals. This way, the glucose will enter the muscles (reducing blood sugar levels in the process) without needing insulin.

Activity is good for the whole body because it:

Walking briskly for thirty minutes five times a week has been nationally adopted as the minimum requirement for healthy benefits. Thirty minutes spread over the day is equally beneficial and activity within your daily routine can also burn calories and improve metabolic function, such as your body's response to insulin.

SELF-HELP

Stress Management. Stress has a part to play in diabetes, both in the inception of Type 2 and in terms of diabetes management. People who suffer from diabetes and who undergo emotional stress such as anxiety or depression tend to have poor glucose control, making them more susceptible to long-term physical complications such as eye, kidney or nerve disorders. Stress management is therefore very important in the management of diabetes. Patients with Type 2 diabetes who incorporate stress management techniques into their routine care can significantly reduce their average blood glucose levels.

Stress management techniques such as instructions on how to identify everyday life stressors and how to respond to them with progressive muscle relaxation and breathing exercises have been shown in studies to reduce the HbA1C score by 0.5% and the blood glucose level by 1% or more.[63] Although this doesn't sound like much, even a 0.5% reduction in HbA1C levels has been shown to produce a significant decrease in diabetic complications.

Acupuncture. The Chinese have long used acupuncture in the treatment of diabetes. Apparently it stimulates the pancreas to make insulin; it increases the number of insulin receptors and it speeds up the body's use of glucose[64]. It often also results in weight loss.

Mind/body techniques, such as thermal biofeedback, have been shown to improve peripheral circulation, pain, neuropathy, ulcers, walking ability and quality of life in people with diabetes.[65]

Sleep. Over time, sleeping five hours or less or nine hours or more each night may increase your risk of developing diabetes. After following more than 70,000 diabetes-free women for a 10-year period, researchers found that women who slept five hours or less every night were 34 percent more likely to develop diabetes symptoms than women who slept for seven or eight hours each night[66]. Comparatively, women who slept nine hours or more each night were 35 percent more likely to develop diabetes symptoms. During the course of the study, which began in 1986, 1,969 women developed diabetes and most showed symptoms of the condition. Researchers were not certain why sleeping too much or too little might be linked to diabetes, though one theory involves leptin, a hormone that may play a role in signaling the body to stop eating. Too little sleep may reduce levels of leptin, possibly causing people to gain weight and develop diabetes. Too much sleep may increase diabetes risk because people who sleep a lot may have sleep apnea, a condition that prevents restful sleep and causes them to sleep more overall due to feeling tired. Independently, sleep apnea may also increase diabetes risk.

Hot Baths. Extraordinary as it may seem, having hot baths may help reduce blood glucose levels. As heat increases metabolism, it also speeds up glucose regulation. A recent study found that subjects who took a 30-minute hot bath every day for 3 weeks lowered their blood glucose levels and lost weight into the bargain.[67]

Relaxation and Laughter. People with Type 2 diabetes may be better able to process sugar from meals if they laugh, according to a small study. Researchers are not certain why laughter appears to reduce blood sugar, but suggested that it might increase the consumption of energy by using the abdominal muscles, or might affect the neuroendocrine system, which controls glucose levels in the blood.[68]

BREAKFASTS

APPLE, PEAR AND TOFU SMOOTHIE

Protein 20%
Carbohydrate 48%
Fat 32%

GI: medium
GL: medium

Smoothies are a great way to start the day, particularly if you are in a hurry, as they only take a few minutes to make. If you are using flax seed, this smoothie thickens on standing, so it needs to be drunk straight away.

1 tbsp	Mixed seeds, e.g. sesame, sunflower, flax seed	1 tbsp
1	Small apple	1
1	Small ripe pear	1
90 g	Tofu, drained and cut into small cubes	3 oz
170 ml	Soya or rice milk	6 fl oz
	A few drops of pure vanilla extract	

Grind the seeds in an electric grinder. Quarter and core the fruit but do not peel. Place all ingredients in a blender and blend until smooth.

Serves 1   **Time taken: 10 minutes**

Per serving
Calories 336kcal; Protein 18g; Carbohydrates 43g; Sugar – Total 29g; Dietary Fibre 10g; Fat – Total 12g; Saturated Fat 2g; Vitamin C 12mg; Magnesium 92mg

Apples and pears are particularly good in the morning because they both have a low GI. The seeds and tofu provide protein, so this smoothie is well-balanced.

TROPICAL TOFU SMOOTHIE

Protein 26%
Carbohydrate 34%
Fat 40%

GI: low
GL: low

This smoothie contains even more tofu than the previous one, combined with fruits that are normally considered too high GI for people with diabetes. However, the addition of soy protein mitigates their effect, and the added flax seeds provide valuable soluble fibre. The end result is an almost perfectly balanced breakfast.

2 tbsp	Flax seeds	2 tbsp
175 g	Tofu, drained and cut into small cubes	6 oz
300 ml	Soya or rice milk	1/2 pint
1	Small, ripe papaya, peeled and chopped	1
1/2	Mango, peeled and cubed	1/2

Grind the seeds in an electric grinder. Place all ingredients in a blender and blend until smooth.

Serves 2   **Time taken: 5 minutes**

Per serving
Calories 263kcal; Protein 18g; Carbohydrates 23g; Sugar – Total 13g; Dietary Fibre 7g; Fat – Total 12g; Saturated Fat 2g; Vitamin C 62mg; Magnesium 100mg

Papayas provide valuable amounts of vitamins C and E, both of which are important antioxidants. Mangoes are one of the very best sources of antioxidant carotenes, and all tropical fruit are rich sources of minerals as they are usually grown on mineral-rich soils.

OAT AND CITRUS SMOOTHIE

Protein 16%   GI: low
Carbohydrate 74%   GL: medium
Fat 10%

The oats for this smoothie should be soaked overnight to make them more digestible. But if you forget to soak them, use 1¹/₂ tbsp and soak for a few minutes. A spoonful of ground mixed seeds is a good addition.

1 tbsp	Rolled oats	1 tbsp
2 tbsp	Oat milk or water	2 tbsp
1	Orange, rind and juice	1
¹/₂	Grapefruit	¹/₂
150 g	Live natural yoghurt	5 oz
	Cinnamon	

Soak the oats overnight in the oat milk or water. In the morning, finely grate the rind from the orange and squeeze out the juice. Squeeze the grapefruit. Put the soaked oats in the blender with the orange and grapefruit juice, orange rind and the yoghurt. Blend until smooth and serve with a dusting of cinnamon.

Serves 1   **Time taken: 10 minutes plus soaking**

Per serving
Calories 286kcal; Protein 12g; Carbohydrates 57g; Sugar – Total 20g; Dietary Fibre 10g; Fat – Total 4g; Saturated Fat 2g; Vitamin C 161mg; Magnesium 52mg

Oats are one of the few readily available sources of chromium in our modern diet. We need chromium to help us metabolise the carbohydrate in our food. Grapefruit and oranges are both low GI, and less than half a teaspoon of cinnamon per day has been found in one study to reduce blood glucose levels by 20% in people with Type 2 diabetes.

APRICOT, SOYA AND PLUM SMOOTHIE

Protein 12%
Carbohydrate 60%
Fat 28%

GI: low
GL: low

Apricots, plums and soya milk are all low GI (soya milk is 43), so this smoothie should help you control your blood glucose. You could substitute live dairy yoghurt if you prefer.

5	Dried apricots	5
2 tbsp	Soya milk	2 tbsp
150 g	Soya yoghurt	5 oz
2	Plums, halved and stoned	2
1 tbsp	Sunflower seeds, ground	1 tbsp

Soak the dried apricots in water overnight, then chop roughly. Place in the blender, together with the soya milk, yoghurt, stoned plums and ground sunflower seeds. Blend until smooth.

Serves 1   **Time taken: 5 minutes plus soaking**

Per serving
Calories 321kcal; Protein 12g; Carbohydrates 45g; Sugar – Total 28g; Dietary Fibre 5g; Fat – Total 12g; Saturated Fat 1g; Vitamin C 17mg; Magnesium 16mg

I have included this smoothie because it contains a range of nutrients, including potassium in the apricots to help regularise blood pressure and vitamin E from the sunflower seeds. Vitamin E is important for people with diabetes as it helps to protect the kidneys.

RAINBOW FRUIT SALAD

Protein 7%   GI: low
Carbohydrate 87%   GL: very low
Fat 6%

*Here I've combined all the most colourful fruit I can think of.
It isn't just that colourful fruits are good to look at – the deeper the
colour the more bioflavonoids they contain, and the more
antioxidant properties they have. Kiwi fruit are a useful source of
vitamin E.*

110 g	Strawberries	4 oz
2	Kiwi fruit	2
60 g	Blueberries	2 oz
4	Fresh apricots	4
60 g	Black seedless grapes	2 oz

Wash all the fruit. Hull the strawberries, cutting in half or quarters
if they are very large. Peel and slice the kiwi fruit. Quarter the
apricots and remove the stones. Cut the grapes in half if large.
Place all the fruit in a bowl and moisten with apple or orange juice
if desired.

Serves 2   **Time taken: 15 minutes**

Per serving
**Calories 123kcal; Protein 2g; Carbohydrates 30g; Sugar – Total
23g; Dietary Fibre 6g; Fat – Total 1g; Saturated Fat 0g; Vitamin
C 99mg; Magnesium 36mg**

> The strawberries can be replaced with raspberries in season.
> Other fruit can be added, but keep a good mix of colours to
> make the fruit salad really appetising. As with any fruit, serving
> it on its own for breakfast would raise the blood glucose too
> high, so accompany with yoghurt and some ground seeds, and
> follow with rye toast or oatcakes.

MARION'S BREAKFAST

Protein 9%   GI: medium
Carbohydrate 79%   GL: low
Fat 12%

Marion is a friend of mine who runs a wonderful bed and breakfast in Aberdovey on the west coast of Wales. This is the breakfast she has every morning before tackling the fry-ups her customers often prefer.

1	Cooking apple	1
1 tbsp	Sultanas	1 tbsp
1 tbsp	Concentrated apple juice	1 tbsp
1 tbsp	Jumbo oats	1 tbsp
2 tsp	Flax seeds	2 tsp
2 tbsp	Apple juice	2 tbsp
	To serve: live yoghurt	

First, make an apple purée: peel and chop the apple roughly, and stew in a tablespoonful of water together with the sultanas until the apple is tender and soft. Stir to make a purée, and sweeten with a little concentrated apple juice. Leave to cool overnight.

The next morning, soak the oats and flax seed in apple juice for 10 minutes or so. Top the oat/flax seed mixture with apple and sultana purée, and serve with live yoghurt.

Serves 1   **Time taken: 15 minutes preparation plus 10 minutes soaking**

Per serving
Calories 286kcal; Protein 7g; Carbohydrates 60g; Sugar – Total 41g; Dietary Fibre 5g; Fat – Total 4g; Saturated Fat 1g; Vitamin C 9mg; Magnesium 28mg

Oats are good for the health of the arteries. The soluble fibre they contain helps to reduce harmful levels of cholesterol in the blood. Jumbo oats are particularly valuable for people with diabetes as they have been minimally processed and therefore they take longer to digest than quick-cooking porridge oats.

OAT AND ALMOND MUESLI

Protein 13%
Carbohydrate 49%
Fat 38%

GI: low
GL: low

It's useful to have some muesli on hand for those days when you are short of time. It is important to soak the muesli, as this makes it more digestible and releases the protein in the oats, nuts and seeds. However, if you forget to soak it the night before, even a few minutes of soaking helps to break down the fibre.

1 lb	Rolled oats	450 g
110 g	Sunflower seeds	4 oz
225 g	Raw almonds, chopped	8 oz
90 g	Sesame seeds, lightly crushed	3 oz
225 g	Unsulphured apricots, chopped	8 oz
110 g	Raisins	4 oz

Simply mix all the ingredients together and store in an airtight container.

To serve, soak about 3 oz/90 g of muesli per serving overnight in an equal volume of water. In the morning, drain off any excess water and serve with soya, nut or rice milk and grated apple on top.

Makes 12 servings　　　　**Time taken: 15 minutes plus soaking**

Per serving
Calories 400kcal; Protein 14g; Carbohydrates 50g; Sugar – Total 16g; Dietary Fibre 8g; Fat – Total 18g; Saturated Fat 2g; Vitamin C 3mg; Magnesium 113mg

Oats are a great source of soluble fibre. One serving of this muesli also contains 5 mcg of chromium, a hard-to-get mineral which is good for keeping blood sugar levels even throughout the morning. The combination of almonds and oats provides an excellent source of magnesium, needed by diabetics for healthy insulin production.

RASPBERRY MUESLI SUNDAE

Protein 16%   GI: low
Carbohydrate 52%   GL: low
Fat 32%

This lovely summery breakfast can be made the night before for a quick getaway next morning. If you don't have raspberries, try other berries such as blueberries or sliced strawberries, or a mixture. There is an unsweetened mixture of frozen 'forest fruits' available in the supermarkets which, when thawed, works very well when berries are out of season.

110 g	Fresh or frozen thawed raspberries	4 oz
150 g	Natural live yoghurt	5 oz
90 g	Oat and almond muesli (see page 51)	3 oz

Put a tablespoon of raspberries into each of two glass dishes or tall glasses. Top each serving of raspberries with a spoonful of yoghurt. Sprinkle a layer of oat and almond muesli on to each serving. Continue the layers until all the ingredients have been used up. Top each serving with a whole raspberry, and refrigerate overnight.
Serves 2   **Time taken: 5 minutes**

Per serving
Calories 266kcal; Protein 11g; Carbohydrates 36g; Sugar – Total 10mg; Dietary Fibre 8g; Fat – Total 10g; Saturated Fat 2g; Vitamin C 16mg; Magnesium 62mg

Raspberries contain a little iron together with a lot of vitamin C, which helps your body absorb the iron. Berries cause a slow increase in blood glucose which helps to lead to a feeling of fullness and does not lead to a large release of insulin.

YOGHURT CHEESE WITH APRICOTS AND WALNUTS

Protein 12%   GI: low
Carbohydrate 76%   GL: medium
Fat 12%

Yoghurt cheese, which is simply strained natural yoghurt, is a good way to get some quality protein for breakfast. The texture is like that of a soft cheese, and it can be used in savoury and sweet dishes. Its taste is a little sharp, which is why I've included some honey in the recipe, but you may find you don't need the honey.

150 g	Natural live yoghurt	5 oz
90 g	Unsulphured dried apricots	3 oz
2 tsp	Honey (optional)	2 tsp
2 tsp	Walnuts, chopped	2 tsp
	Ground cinnamon, for serving	

Spoon the yoghurt into a fine-meshed sieve over a bowl and leave to drain overnight in the refrigerator. Put the apricots into a small saucepan, cover with cold water and simmer for 10 minutes or so. Leave covered with water overnight.

Next morning, drain the apricots, chop roughly, and put into a bowl with the honey.

Discard the liquid which has drained off the yoghurt, and add the yoghurt to the apricot and honey mixture, together with the chopped walnuts. Spoon into two individual serving bowls and sprinkle with cinnamon.

Serves 2   **Time taken: 5 minutes plus overnight soaking**

Per serving
Calories 212kcal; Protein 7g; Carbohydrates 41g; Sugar – Total 24g; Dietary Fibre 3g; Fat – Total 3g; Saturated Fat 1g; Vitamin C 8mg; Magnesium 4mg

Dried apricots have a GI of 30, which is quite low. They are an excellent source of beta-carotene and very high in potassium. They are quite high in fructose, which helps to lower their GI value. Although there are concerns about refined fructose (see page 32), the fructose naturally occurring in fruits is perfectly fine for people with diabetes.

BREAKFAST BARLEY WITH MOLASSES AND PEARS

Protein 7%
Carbohydrate 85%
Fat 8%

GI: low
GL: low

Barley is an underrated grain, in my opinion, usually only making its appearance in soups or stews. It makes a very tasty and sustaining breakfast on a cold morning.

6 tbsp	Pearl barley	6 tbsp
600 ml	Cold water	1 pint
2	Pears	2
2 tbsp	Blackstrap molasses	2 tbsp
	Soya milk or rice milk, to serve	
2 tsp	Sunflower seeds	2 tsp

Place the barley in a saucepan and cover with the water. Bring to the boil, then lower the heat and cook, covered, until soft to the bite. This will take 45-60 minutes, and is better done the night before you want to eat it. Cool, covered, overnight. In the morning, add the milk of your choice and the molasses, and bring to simmering point. Cook for a few minutes until heated through, then stir in the chopped pear before serving. Sprinkle with sunflower seeds.

Serves 2

Time taken: 1 hour the day before plus 5 minutes reheating

Per serving
Calories 254kcal; Protein 5g; Carbohydrates 57g; Sugar – Total 20g; Dietary Fibre 9g; Fat – Total 2g; Saturated Fat 0g; Vitamin C 6mg; Magnesium 66mg

Pearl barley is unusual in that, although it is a relatively refined grain, it has a very low GI, probably because it is high in soluble fibre. The sunflower seeds provide a useful amount of vitamin E.

CHICKPEA AND TOMATO FRITTATA

Protein 20%
Carbohydrate 30%
Fat 50%

GI: low
GL: low

I'm sure this isn't an authentic Italian frittata, but it came about when I was trying to think of ways to include pulses in the breakfast menu. Pulses such as chickpeas are so good for moderating the blood glucose level, as they provide ready mixed protein and complex carbohydrate, that people with diabetes should incorporate them into their daily eating pattern whenever possible. This frittata is also good eaten cold for lunch.

225 g	Cooked chickpeas (or one 14 oz/ 400 g can, drained and rinsed)	8 oz
2	Large beefsteak tomatoes, peeled, seeded and diced	2
2 tbsp	Extra virgin olive oil	2 tbsp
6	Organic, free range eggs	6
	Sea salt and freshly ground black pepper	
2 tbsp	Chopped flat-leaf parsley or finely shredded fresh basil	2 tbsp

Beat the eggs with seasoning to taste, and add half the parsley or basil. Heat the olive oil in a large frying pan over gentle heat. Pour the eggs into the pan and then add the chickpeas and diced tomato. Cook until nearly set. If you like your frittata quite firm, preheat the grill while the frittata is cooking, then slip the frying pan under the grill for a minute or two, just to set the top.
Serve hot or at room temperature, cut into wedges, with the remainder of the parsley or basil sprinkled over the top.
Serves 4   **Time taken: 20 minutes**

Per serving
Calories 271kcal; Protein 14g; Carbohydrates 21g; Sugar – Total 4g; Dietary Fibre 5g; Fat – Total 15g; Saturated Fat 3g; Vitamin C 21mg; Magnesium 47mg

Tomatoes are a valuable source of lycopene, a powerful antioxidant especially when cooked, and even more so when accompanied by healthy fats, such as those found in olive oil.

BAKED EGGS WITH MUSHROOMS

Protein 19%
Carbohydrate 5%
Fat 76%

GI: very low
GL: very low

Eggs are a great source of protein for starting the day and keeping your energy levels up. I've baked them on a bed of mushrooms here, but you could substitute lightly cooked spinach or tomatoes if you prefer. Add a teaspoon of miso to each serving for extra flavour and protein. For a balanced meal, precede an egg dish like this with a smoothie or fruit salad.

1 tbsp	Extra virgin olive oil	1 tbsp
60 g	Button mushrooms, sliced	2 oz
	Freshly grated nutmeg	
2 tsp	Miso (optional)	2 tsp
2	Organic, free range eggs	2
	Sea salt and freshly ground black pepper to taste	

Preheat the oven to 200°C/400°F/Gas Mark 6. Lightly grease 2 ramekins and sprinkle each one with nutmeg.

Heat the oil in a small pan, then add the mushrooms. Sautée on a low heat for 5-8 minutes until the juices run. Stir in the miso, if using, and season to taste.

Divide the mushrooms between the ramekins and make a well in each one. Crack an egg into each well. Bake for 10–15 minutes and serve hot.

Serves 2   **Time taken: 25 minutes**

Per serving
Calories 145kcal; Protein 7g; Carbohydrates 2g; Sugar – Total 1g; Dietary Fibre 0g; Fat – Total 12g; Saturated Fat 3g; Vitamin C 1mg; Magnesium 12mg

Do not be alarmed at the apparently high proportion of fat in this recipe, most of which comes from the egg yolk. There's as much monounsaturated fat in an egg as there is saturated fat, and it provides so much else – a useful amount of protein, B vitamins and vitamin E.

WHOLEGRAIN AND SEED MUFFINS

Protein 14%
Carbohydrate 40%
Fat 46%

GI: medium
GL: high

The natural sweetness in these muffins is provided by the sunflower seeds, which are good sources of essential fatty acids, protein and magnesium.

110 g	Rolled oats	4 oz
110 g	Wholemeal flour	4 oz
45 g	Sunflower seeds	1½ oz
2 tbsp	Flax seed	2 tbsp
1½ tsp	Salt-free baking powder	1½ tsp
½ tsp	Bicarbonate of soda	½ tsp
1	Organic, free range egg	1
4 tbsp	Extra virgin olive oil	4 tbsp
125 g	Natural yoghurt or soya yoghurt	4½ oz
2 tbsp	Soya, rice or nut milk	2 tbsp

Preheat oven to 190°C/375°F/Gas Mark 5. Either spray 12 muffin tins with olive oil spray, use non-stick muffin tins, or use paper muffin cases, which don't need oiling.

Mix together the oats, flour, seeds, baking powder and bicarbonate of soda in a large bowl. In a separate bowl, beat together the egg, oil, yoghurt and your chosen milk. Next, add the egg mixture to the dry ingredients, combining the two mixtures with a few swift strokes to form a fairly stiff dough. Spoon into the prepared muffin tins and bake for 15 minutes in the preheated oven.

Leave in the muffin tins for a few minutes before turning out onto a rack to cool.

Makes 12 muffins   **Time taken: 25 minutes**

Per muffin
Calories 149kcals; Protein 5g; Carbohydrates 16g; Dietary Fibre 3g; Sugar – Total 1g; Fat – Total 8g; Saturated Fat 1g; Vitamin C 0mg; Magnesium 40mg

These muffins are high in both calcium and magnesium. They are good on their own, or try them with a pure fruit spread, such as St Dalfour or Meridian.

SNACKS AND DRINKS

QUICK SARDINE PÂTÉ

Protein 43%
Carbohydrate 7%
Fat 50%

GI: low
GL: low

This easy pâté is delicious spread on rye bread or oatcakes. As a variation, try it with other canned fish such as mackerel or pilchards. Smoked mackerel is good too.

1	Tin of sardines packed in olive oil	1
1 tsp	Horseradish sauce	1 tsp
1 tbsp	Finely chopped onion	1 tbsp
1 tsp	Fresh parsley, finely chopped	1 tsp
1 tsp	Fresh lemon juice	1 tsp
	Paprika, to serve	

Drain the sardines and mash them, together with the horseradish, in a small bowl. Add the chopped onion and parsley and season to taste with lemon juice.

Serve on pumpernickel or rye toast with a dusting of paprika on top.

Serves 1   **Time taken: 5 minutes**

Per serving
Calories 137kcals; Protein 14g; Carbohydrates 2g; Dietary Fibre 0g; Sugar – Total 1g; Fat – Total 7g; Saturated Fat 1g; Vitamin C 5mg; Magnesium 26mg

Sardines are a rich source of omega-3 fatty acids, known to help reduce risk of heart disease, high blood pressure, and cancer.

WHITE BEAN AND MINT HUMMUS

Protein 12%   GI: medium
Carbohydrate 46%   GL: low
Fat 42%

This is a delicious variation on traditional hummus, which is made with chickpeas. Do not be put off by the large amount of garlic in this recipe – roasting it first imparts a mellow flavour which is not strong at all. I have suggested canned beans here for convenience, but if you prefer to cook them from scratch, use 100 g/3½ oz dried beans which will yield the right amount of cooked beans for this recipe.

1	Small head of garlic	1
1 tsp	Extra virgin olive oil, for drizzling	1 tsp
2 tsp	Ground cumin	2 tsp
½ tsp	Chilli powder (optional)	½ tsp
1	400 g can of cannellini beans, haricot beans or butter beans, drained and rinsed	1
1	Handful fresh mint leaves, chopped	1
½	Lemon, juice only	½
2 tbsp	Extra virgin olive oil	2 tbsp
	Sea salt and freshly ground black pepper to taste	

First, roast the garlic. Preheat the oven to 180°C/350°F/Gas Mark 4. Cut the top off the head of garlic, place on a baking tray, drizzle with a little olive oil and roast for 35-40 minutes or until soft. Leave to cool, then pop the garlic cloves out of their skins. Even if you don't use all the garlic, it is a good idea to roast it whole – single cloves usually dry up too much when roasted. Any unused roasted garlic cloves make a tasty addition to a sauce or salad dressing.

Dry roast the cumin and chilli powder, if using, in a small pan over medium heat until the cumin gives off its aroma.

Place the garlic cloves, drained beans, chopped mint, lemon juice, olive oil and toasted spices in a food processor and process until smooth. Season to taste and serve at room temperature as a spread or dip.

Serves 2   Time taken: 50 minutes

Per serving
Calories 329kcals; Protein 10g; Carbohydrates 38g; Dietary Fibre 9g; Sugar – Total 1g; Fat – Total 15g; Saturated Fat 2g; Vitamin C 17mg; Magnesium 13mg

SPICY CHICKPEA SNACKS

Protein 21%   GI: low
Carbohydrate 65%   GL: low
Fat 14%

These are terribly easy, and good to have on hand to serve with drinks. Warning – the chickpeas have a tendency to jump about or even explode if the oven is too hot, so if this starts to happen, remove the tray from the oven, cool it a little, then return the tray to finish cooking at a lower temperature.

450 g	Dried chickpeas	1 lb
½ tsp	Sea salt	½ tsp
¼ tsp	Cayenne pepper, or to taste	¼ tsp

Preheat the oven to 180°C/350°F/Gas Mark 4.

Soak the chickpeas overnight in plenty of cold water. The next day, drain thoroughly.

Spread the chickpeas in a single layer on a baking tray or trays. Bake in the preheated oven until crisp and shrunk again to their original size (about 45 minutes).

Toss with sea salt and cayenne pepper while still hot. Taste as you do this as a heavy hand with the seasoning could ruin the effect. Store in an airtight tin and serve cold as a snack with drinks.

Variation: These are also delicious tossed with curry powder. Whichever seasoning you choose, try sprinkling the chickpeas with a few drops of olive oil when you remove them from the oven.

Serves 16   Time taken: 50 minutes plus overnight soaking

Per serving
Calories 96kcal; Protein 5g; Carbohydrates 16g; Dietary Fibre 4g; Sugar – Total 1g; Fat – Total 2g; Saturated Fat 0g; Vitamin C 1mg; Magnesium 28mg

Chickpeas have a low GI – the average of four different studies was 28. Like other pulses, they are digested slowly and are therefore very valuable to people with diabetes. Over the long term they may help to improve blood glucose control.

TAMARI SEEDS

Protein 15%
Carbohydrate 14%
Fat 71%

GI: low
GL: low

These seeds are quite salty owing to the tamari sauce, so if you're using them as a nibble with a drink, have some water as well. This saltiness is the natural flavour of tamari, which is a wheat-free, naturally fermented Japanese soy sauce. This treatment can also be given to soaked soya beans, but they will need longer in the oven – about 20 minutes.

250 g	Sunflower seeds	8¹/₂ oz
250 g	Pumpkin seeds	8¹/₂ oz
4 tbsp	Tamari	4 tbsp

Preheat the oven to 180°C/350°F/Gas Mark 4.

Mix the seeds together in a large bowl and toss with the tamari so that the seeds are well coated. Spread out on baking trays in a single layer and roast for 10-15 minutes, turning from time to time, until the seeds are golden brown. Cool and serve as a snack with drinks.

Serves 16   **Time taken: 20 minutes**

Per serving
Calories 178kcals; Protein 7g; Carbohydrates 7g; Dietary Fibre 2g; Sugar – Total 1g; Fat – Total 15g; Saturated Fat 2g; Vitamin C 1mg; Magnesium 104mg

Pumpkin seeds have many virtues, one of which is their high magnesium content. Magnesium is an important mineral for people with diabetes as it can help promote healthy insulin production. It can also reduce the craving for sweet foods, thus helping to prevent Type 2 diabetes.

FRUIT AND NUT TRUFFLES

Protein 8%   GI: low
Carbohydrate 41%   GL: low
Fat 51%

Sometimes you just want a sweet treat, and that's where these come in. Dates are high GI, so they should only be regarded as something to have after a balanced meal rather than eaten on their own. And here their effect on blood sugar is mitigated by the fat and protein in the nuts and seeds.

90 g	Dates, stoned	3 oz
90 g	Raisins	3 oz
3 tbsp	Organic cocoa powder, such as Green & Black's	3 tbsp
90 g	Walnuts, chopped	3 oz
75 g	Sunflower seeds	2½ oz

Place the dates and raisins in a small saucepan with a little water. Bring to a gentle simmer for about 5 minutes, just to soften them. Drain and cool. Place the dates, raisins, 2 tablespoons of the cocoa powder, walnuts and sunflower seeds in a food processor, and process until everything is finely chopped and the mixture adheres into a large ball. With your hands, form the mixture into 24 small balls. Roll in the last tablespoonful of cocoa powder. Place truffles in paper cases and refrigerate for a few hours. Serve chilled.

Makes 24 truffles   **Time taken: 20 minutes**

Per truffle
Calories 66kcals; Protein 2g; Carbohydrates 7g; Dietary Fibre 1g; Sugar – Total 5g; Fat – Total 4g; Saturated Fat 0g; Vitamin C 0mg; Magnesium 16mg

If you cannot tolerate cocoa – for instance, if you suffer from migraines – substitute carob powder for the cocoa powder. Carob is a very good source of calcium and has a delicious taste, often indistinguishable from cocoa.

DRINKS

JUICES

Vegetable juices are an excellent source of vitamins and minerals and other phyto-nutrients that have been shown to combat disease. Because juices are raw, the vitamin C and other water-soluble vitamins and enzymes that are largely lost in cooking are still intact. Juices are easily absorbed and therefore offer instant energy without pushing up your blood glucose. I don't recommend pure fruit juices for people with diabetes, as these contain concentrated fructose and may cause a rapid rise in blood glucose, though adding a little low GI fruit to a mixed vegetable juice enhances the flavour and should not have too great an effect on blood sugar. The juice of sweeter vegetables, such as carrot and beetroot, should be treated with caution and only drunk mixed with that of green leafy vegetables such as spinach or watercress.

The preparation of fruit and vegetables for juicing will depend on the kind of juicer you have. All produce should be well washed (and peeled unless it is organic) and cut up to fit the feeding tube of your juicer. If you are using a centrifugal juicer, the juice should be drunk immediately as it will deteriorate quickly. The more expensive masticator type of juicer makes better juice which lasts longer. I have not given a method for the first four of these recipes as it is basically the same for any juice. Just prepare the produce, put it through the juicer and enjoy.

Here are some ideas, but feel free to make up your own combinations. Use organic produce whenever possible to avoid chemical residues which cannot be washed off. If you can't get organic vegetables, peel or wash in water acidulated with a spoonful of cider vinegar.

SPINACH, CARROT AND BEETROOT JUICE

Protein 10%
Carbohydrate 87%
Fat 3%

GI: medium
GL: low

This juice is utterly delicious and a great way to introduce yourself to vegetable juices.

1 handful	Spinach leaves	1 handful
2	Large carrots, peeled if not organic	2
1	Small cooking apple, quartered and cored	1
1	Small raw beetroot, scrubbed, with leaves if possible	1

Serves 1   Time taken: 5 minutes

Per serving
Calories 163kcals; Protein 5g; Carbohydrates 40g; Dietary Fibre 0g; Sugar – Total 28g; Fat – Total 1g; Saturated Fat 0g; Vitamin C 39mg; Magnesium 88mg

Lots of valuable nutrients here: the spinach provides vitamin C, folic acid and vitamin K, the carrots provide a huge amount of beta-carotene and some vitamin C, the beetroot provides folic acid and the apples vitamin C. All these nutrients are needed for bone health, skin health, heart health and immunity.

MORE THAN TOMATO JUICE

Protein 16%   GI: low
Carbohydrate 73%   GL: low
Fat 11%

The addition of watercress makes this juice delightfully peppery.

5	Ripe medium-sized tomatoes	5
1	Bunch watercress, well washed	1
2	Sticks of celery	2

Serves 1   Time taken: 5 minutes

Per serving
Calories 148kcals; Protein 7g; Carbohydrates 32g; Dietary Fibre
0g; Sugar – Total 18g; Fat – Total 2g; Saturated Fat 0g; Vitamin
C 187mg; Magnesium 87mg

> Tomatoes contain an antioxidant called lycopene, good for
> protecting against free radicals. It is especially important for
> people with diabetes to eat a diet high in antioxidants as they
> tend to have low antioxidant status and are therefore more
> vulnerable to free radical damage.

GARDENER'S TONIC

Protein 13%   GI: medium
Carbohydrate 81%   GL: low
Fat 6%

*This juice gets its name because you could grow all its ingredients in
your own garden, and it's a wonderful pick-me-up tonic.
The cucumber adds a surprisingly strong flavour.*

1	Large leaf of dark green or Savoy cabbage	1
1	Handful of spinach	1
3	Carrots, peeled unless organic	3
½	Cucumber, peeled unless organic	½
½	Red or yellow pepper, deseeded	½

Serves 1   Time taken: 5 minutes

Per serving
Calories 143kcals; Protein 5g; Carbohydrates 33g; Dietary Fibre
0g; Sugar – Total 16g; Fat – Total 1g; Saturated Fat 0g; Vitamin
C 267mg; Magnesium 85mg

> There is a stunning amount of vitamin C in this juice, mostly
> due to the red pepper, provided it was picked when ripe and has
> not been stored for too long. Peppers are actually one of the
> best sources of vitamin C, but this vitamin is easily damaged by
> light, air and storage, so buy your vegetables as fresh as
> possible, consume them quickly and don't cut them up too
> soon before eating.

BROCCOLI, TOMATO AND CUCUMBER JUICE

Protein 18%
Carbohydrate 72%
Fat 10%

GI: low
GL: low

Broccoli makes a strong-tasting juice which is best mixed in a ratio of about 1:4 with the juice of milder tasting vegetables, but its nutritional benefits are so good it is worth getting used to the taste. I cook the broccoli heads and use the thick stems either sliced raw in salads or in juices like this one.

4	Ripe medium tomatoes	4
2	Broccoli stems	2
¹/₂	Cucumber, peeled unless organic	¹/₂

Serves 1   Time taken: 5 minutes

Per serving
Calories 141kcals; Protein 7g; Carbohydrates 30g; Dietary Fibre 0g; Sugar – Total 18g; Fat – Total 2g; Saturated Fat 0g; Vitamin C 188mg; Magnesium 68mg

Broccoli is an excellent food for people with diabetes for many reasons, one of which is that it is a good source of vitamin K. Protecting the body from insulin resistance appears to be one of vitamin K's many roles in the body.

GRAPE AND GREEN

Protein 16%   GI: low
Carbohydrate 78%   GL: low
Fat 6%

This odd-sounding mixture comes from Natalie Savona's inspiring
Big Book of Juices and Smoothies. *I would not have thought of*
combining grapefruit and kale, but it works surprisingly well.

1	Grapefruit	1
2	Handfuls of spinach	2
2	Sticks of celery	2
4	Leaves of curly kale	4

First, juice the grapefruit using a citrus juicer. Then put the rest of
the ingredients through the juicer and stir in the grapefruit juice.
Serves 1   **Time taken: 10 minutes**

Per serving
Calories 143kcals; Protein 6g; Carbohydrates 31g; Dietary Fibre
0g; Sugar – Total 20g; Fat – Total 1g; Saturated Fat 0g; Vitamin
C 186mg; Magnesium 126mg

This juice is particularly good for people with diabetes because
grapefruit are low GI. If you can save some of the white pith of
the grapefruit (but not the bitter peel) to put through the juicer,
this will give you a shot of bioflavonoids. The kale and spinach
provide lots of magnesium, an important nutrient for diabetics.

HOT AND COLD BEVERAGES

CAROB, DATE AND ALMOND MILK

Protein 10%
Carbohydrate 40%
Fat 50%

GI: low
GL: low

I love almond milk and often have it on cereal or porridge. Adding carob and dates is simply gilding the lily. If it is too much bother to make your own almond milk, you can purchase it from a good health food shop and blend it with the dates and carob powder. This drink is also delicious made with soaked dried figs.

45 g	Whole almonds, soaked overnight	1½ oz
3	Stoned dates, soaked overnight	3
175 ml	Filtered or bottled water	6 fl oz
2 tbsp	Carob powder	2 tbsp
	A few drops of almond extract	

Blend all the ingredients in a blender on high speed until smooth and creamy. To separate the liquid from the almond skins and pulp, press through a fine metal sieve set over a bowl, using the back of a spoon. Alternatively, you can line the sieve with a piece of clean muslin. This has the advantage that you can squeeze the muslin with your hands to extract as much milk as possible. Serve at room temperature or chilled, and shake well before serving.

Serves 1   **Time taken: 15 minutes**

Per serving
Calories 355kcals; Protein 10g; Carbohydrates 38g; Dietary Fibre 6g; Sugar – Total 18g; Fat – Total 22g; Saturated Fat 2g; Vitamin C 0mg; Magnesium 17mg

> Almonds are an excellent addition to the diet for a number of reasons, one of which is that they are the best dietary source of calcium. They are also a rich source of vitamin E, needed especially by people with diabetes.

FRESH GINGER MINT TEA

Protein 17%
Carbohydrate 72%
Fat 11%

GI: low
GL: low

Home made herbal teas are much more vibrant and zingy than those bought in sachets. Try this one in the summer when mint grows like a weed.

5 cm	Piece of fresh root ginger	2 inches
1	Small handful fresh sprigs of mint, washed	1
600 ml	Filtered or bottled water	1 pint

Peel and slice or grate the ginger into a teapot or other heatproof receptacle. Add the sprigs of mint. Boil the water and pour over the ginger and mint. Stir and cover. Leave to steep for at least 5 minutes before straining and drinking hot or warm.

Variation: fresh lemon and ginger tea can be made substituting lemon slices for the mint.

Serves 2 **Time taken: 10 minutes**

Per serving
Calories 5kcals; Protein 0g; Carbohydrates 1g; Dietary Fibre 0g; Sugar – Total 0g; Fat – Total 0g; Saturated Fat 0g; Vitamin C 1mg; Magnesium 8mg

There is some evidence that ginger can help stabilise insulin levels if taken 40 minutes before a meal[69], and this tea is a delightful way to test this theory.

SPICY GINGER AND FENNEL TEA

Protein 13%   GI: low
Carbohydrate 64%   GL: low
Fat 23%

This tea is very soothing to the digestive tract, and is good drunk before, with or after a meal.

5 cm	Piece of fresh root ginger	2 inches
1 tbsp	Fennel seeds	1 tbsp
1	Cinnamon stick	1
2	Cloves	2
600 ml	Filtered or bottled water	1 pint

Peel and grate the ginger. Crush the fennel seeds in a mortar and pestle. Break up the cinnamon stick. Put all the spices in a teapot or other heatproof receptacle. Boil the water and pour over the spices. Stir, cover and allow to stand for 10 minutes. Strain and drink hot.
Serves 2   **Time taken: 15 minutes**

Per serving
Calories 17kcal; Protein 1g; Carbohydrates 3g; Dietary Fibre 0g; Sugar – Total 0g; Fat – Total 0g; Saturated Fat 0g; Vitamin C 1mg; Magnesium 13mg

> Fennel seeds are gently tonic and diuretic. Their main use is for digestive problems, such as poor digestion, bloating, nausea and flatulence. This is a very good tea to drink if you are feeling a bit queasy.

FENUGREEK TEA

Protein 24%   GI: low
Carbohydrate 61%   GL: low
Fat 15%

This tea may be drunk several times a day to help lower blood glucose. If you can't find fenugreek seeds, substitute with powdered fenugreek.

1 tbsp	Fenugreek seed	1 tbsp
600 ml	Filtered or bottled water	1 pint

Soak the seeds in the water for three hours, then strain. Reheat to serve, or drink the tea iced.

Serves 2   **Time taken: 5 minutes plus 3 hours soaking**

Per serving
Calories 36kcals; Protein 3g; Carbohydrates 6g; Dietary Fibre 3g; Sugar – Total 0g; Fat – Total 1g; Saturated Fat 0g; Vitamin C 0mg; Magnesium 24mg

Fenugreek seeds are a traditional Indian remedy, recently confirmed by Western scientists. Studies have shown that active ingredients in the seeds raise HDL (the 'good' cholesterol) and lower blood glucose. The unique dietary fibre composition and high saponin content in fenugreek appears to be responsible for these therapeutic properties.[70]

JUNIPER BERRY WINE

Protein 1%
Carbohydrate 5%
Fat 0%
Alcohol: 94%

GI: high
GL: low

This idea comes from Food is Medicine *by Pierre Jean Cousin, a Frenchman who makes looking after your health sound like going out for a restaurant meal. The recommended dose for people with diabetes is 50 ml per day.*

1	750 ml bottle white wine	1
75 g	Juniper berries, crushed	2¹/₂ oz
2 tsp	Lemon zest from organic lemons	2 tsp

Decant the wine into a container that can be sealed. Add the juniper berries and lemon zest to the wine. Seal tightly and leave for a week. Strain through muslin and store in a tightly sealed bottle.

Makes 15 servings   Time taken: 5 minutes plus 1 week standing

Per serving
Calories 102kcals; Protein 0g; Carbohydrates 1g; Dietary Fibre 0g; Sugar – Total 0g; Fat – Total 0g; Saturated Fat 0g; Vitamin C 1mg; Magnesium 15mg

Juniper was traditionally used in the treatment of diabetes in the days before insulin was available. In a recent study the blood sugar lowering effect of juniper was tested on mice, together with that of various other herbs such as agrimony, alfalfa, coriander, eucalyptus and others. The results suggested that these traditional plant treatments for diabetes, including juniper, could retard the development of diabetes in mice.[71]

SOUPS AND STARTERS

CREAM OF AVOCADO SOUP WITH COCONUT MILK

Protein 8%
Carbohydrate 17%
Fat 75%

GI: low
GL: low

This absurdly easy but sophisticated soup comes from the days I spent cooking on yachts in the Caribbean. It was ideal for catering at sea because it was quick and foolproof. The quantities are not large, but it is very rich, so you don't need much.

2	Large avocados	2
½ tsp	Sea salt	½ tsp
225 ml	Coconut milk	8 fl oz
1	Lime, juice only	1
425 ml	Vegetable stock (see page 158)	15 fl oz
1 tbsp	Dry sherry (optional)	1 tbsp
	Dash of hot sauce, such as Tabasco	
	Slices of lime and coriander leaves, for garnish	

Cut the avocados in half. Remove the seeds and scoop out the flesh. Place the avocado flesh, salt, coconut milk, and lime juice in a blender or food processor. Blend to a smooth purée. Heat the vegetable stock to boiling point. With the machine running, slowly add the hot stock to the purée. Stir in the sherry, if using, and a dash of hot sauce to taste. This soup may be served hot or cold.

If serving hot, heat but do not let it boil. If serving cold, refrigerate for several hours and serve in cold bowls. Garnish each serving with a thin slice of lime and a couple of whole coriander leaves.

Serves 4   **Time taken: 10 minutes**

Per serving
Calories 269kcal; Protein 4g; Carbohydrates 12g; Sugar – Total 3g; Dietary Fibre 9g; Fat – Total 24g; Saturated Fat 13g; Vitamin C 9mg; Magnesium 34mg

I'm glad to say that avocados are back on the menu these days, having fallen out of favour. The fat they contain is nearly all oleic acid, a monounsaturated fat, and they are a very good source of vitamin E, an important nutrients for people with diabetes.

BROCCOLI SOUP WITH HORSERADISH

Protein 11%
Carbohydrate 40%
Fat 49%

GI: medium
GL: low

The horseradish in this soup provides a pleasant 'bite'. If you can't find fresh horseradish, substitute 2-3 teaspoons of creamed horseradish and omit the yoghurt. You could try this soup using cauliflower instead of broccoli, as cauliflower would stand up to the horseradish equally well, and has a similar nutritional profile to broccoli.

2 tbsp	Extra virgin olive oil	2 tbsp
1	Small onion, peeled and finely chopped	1
110 g	Potato, peeled and diced	4 oz
340 g	Broccoli, roughly chopped	12 oz
1 litre	Vegetable stock (see page 158)	1³/₄ pints
1	Organic lime, juice and finely grated zest	1
1 tbsp	Fresh parsley, chopped	1 tbsp
1 tbsp	Fresh chives, chopped	1 tbsp
2 tbsp	Live natural yoghurt	2 tbsp
2 tsp	Freshly grated horseradish	2 tsp
Sea salt and freshly ground black pepper to taste		

Heat the oil in a large pan and sauté the chopped onion and potato over gentle heat until softened but not brown. Add the vegetable stock, lime zest and juice, bring to the boil and simmer for 30 minutes, until the vegetables are soft.

Meanwhile, steam the broccoli in another pot until just tender but still green – about 8 minutes. As soon as it is cooked, plunge straight away into cold water to set the colour. Drain well and set aside.

When the potato and onion mixture is cooked, take off the heat, cool a little and then blend to a smooth consistency in the blender or food processor. Add the cooked broccoli and blend again briefly – there should still be recognizable pieces of broccoli. Return to a clean saucepan and stir in the chopped herbs, yoghurt, grated horseradish and seasoning to taste. Reheat without boiling, check seasoning and serve piping hot in heated bowls.

Serves 4   **Time taken: 50 minutes**

Per serving
Calories 150kcal; Protein 4g; Carbohydrates 15g; Sugar – Total 4g; Dietary Fibre 5g; Fat – Total 8g; Saturated Fat 1g; Vitamin C 80mg; Magnesium 29mg

I have come to regard broccoli as something of a superfood, and I think we should all be eating it at least once a day. It is ranked first in the US National Cancer Institute's list of all-round anti-cancer vegetables as it is rich in several potential anticancer substances such as indoles, glucosinolates, beta-carotene and vitamin C. Not only that, but it is one of the richest sources of iron in the vegetable world and contains a significant amount of magnesium.

GAZPACHO WITH AUBERGINE CROÛTONS

Protein 8%
Carbohydrate 34%
Fat 58%

GI: low
GL: low

This is a raw soup. There are huge advantages to eating raw food – none of the nutrients are lost in cooking, and the plant enzymes are for the most part still intact. Gazpacho is normally bulked out with white breadcrumbs, but I use ground almonds to boost the protein and fatty acid content and reduce the carbohydrate load.

4 tbsp	Ground almonds	4 tbsp
2	Garlic cloves, peeled and crushed	2
1 tbsp	Red wine vinegar	1 tbsp
1 tbsp	Extra virgin olive oil	1 tbsp
1	Green pepper, coarsely chopped	1
1	Onion, coarsely chopped	1
5	Very ripe tomatoes, peeled, seeded and coarsely chopped	5
1	Cucumber, peeled and coarsely chopped	1
1 tbsp	Tomato purée	1 tbsp
	Sea salt, to taste	
	For the aubergine croûtons:	
2 tbsp	Extra virgin olive oil	2 tbsp
1/2	Medium aubergine	1/2

Put the ground almonds and garlic in a small bowl. Add the vinegar and olive oil. Mix well, cover and set aside for a couple of hours to let the flavours combine. Put the green pepper, onion, tomatoes, cucumber, tomato purée and almond mixture in a blender or food processor. Process briefly, until vegetables are just chopped. You may have to do this in two batches. Transfer the mixture to a large chilled bowl and stir in enough very cold water to give the soup a creamy consistency. Season to taste and refrigerate until ready to serve.

To make the croûtons, heat the olive oil in a frying pan or wok over high heat. Add the aubergine cubes and stir fry over high heat until they are browned. Drain well on kitchen paper.

It makes an interesting contrast with the chilled soup if you can serve the croûtons very hot, but if not, room temperature is fine.

Serves 4   **Time taken: 20 minutes plus 2 hours resting**

Per serving
Calories 208kcal; Protein 4g; Carbohydrates 19g; Sugar – Total 9g; Dietary Fibre 5g; Fat – Total 14g; Saturated Fat 2g;Vitamin C 62mg; Magnesium 48mg

This soup depends largely on the quality of the tomatoes used. It is worth searching out tomatoes that have been ripened on the vine, thus allowing them to develop not only a depth of flavour but also more nutritional value. Fruit and vegetables that have been harvested before they are ripe are nutritionally depleted.

BUTTER BEAN SOUP WITH PARSLEY PESTO

Protein 20%	GI: low
Carbohydrate 52%	GL: low
Fat 28%	

I've used butter beans in this soup, but you could substitute any pale coloured bean, such as white haricot beans, cannellini beans or flageolet beans. I love the contrast of the white soup and the dark green pesto, not to mention the delicious flavour. The addition of ginger seems to help counteract the unfortunate tendency of beans to cause flatulence in some people.

225 g	Butter beans, soaked overnight in water	8 oz
1	Thumb-sized piece of root ginger, peeled	1
2 tbsp	Extra virgin olive oil	2 tbsp

1	Large onion, chopped	1
2 sticks	Celery, chopped	2 sticks
1 litre	Chicken stock (see page 159)	1¾ pints
	Sea salt and freshly ground black pepper to taste	
	For the parsley pesto:	1 tsp
1	Small bunch flat leaf parsley, roughly chopped	1
1	Clove garlic, crushed	1
2 tbsp	Parmesan cheese, finely grated	2 tbsp
2 tbsp	Extra virgin olive oil	2 tbsp
	Sea salt and freshly ground black pepper to taste	
	Lemon juice, to taste	

Drain the butter beans and cover with clean cold water. Add the ginger, bring to the boil and cook at a rolling boil for 10 minutes, skimming off any foam as it boils. Reduce the heat, cover and simmer until the beans are tender. This depends on their age, and can take anything from 1-2 hours. When they are soft, remove from the heat, drain the beans and discard the piece of ginger.

Heat the olive oil in a large pan and sauté the onion and celery over gentle heat until softened but not browned. Add the drained beans, chicken stock and seasoning, bring to the boil and cook for another 30-40 minutes until the beans and vegetables are really soft. Cool a little, then blend in the blender or food processor, and check for seasoning. Return the soup to the pan and reheat.

While the soup is cooking, make the parsley pesto: place the chopped parsley into a food processor with the garlic and Parmesan. Process until smooth. With the motor still running, slowly add the olive oil and a squeeze of lemon juice. Season with salt and pepper.

Serve the soup very hot with a swirl of parsley pesto in each bowl.

Variations: The pesto can be made with any strongly flavoured herb, such as coriander or the traditional basil.

Serves 4   Time taken: 3 hours

Per serving
Calories 282kcal; Protein 14g; Carbohydrates 37g; Sugar – Total 8g; Dietary Fibre 12g; Fat – Toal 9g; Saturated Fat 2g; Vitamin C 26mg; Magnesium 80mg

At 31, the GI of butter beans is very low. They have other beneficial properties, too. Like all pulses, they are a combination of protein and carbohydrate and an extremely good source of soluble fibre. This means that they are digested slowly and so are naturally good for balancing blood glucose.

JUNE'S SPICY CHANA DAL SOUP

Protein 15%   GI: very low
Carbohydrate 46%   GL: low
Fat 39%

This soup comes from June Marriott, my sister-in-law and a gifted cook. She makes it with chickpeas, but chana dal cooks in the same way as chickpeas and tastes quite similar whilst having a far lower GI, so it is invaluable for people with diabetes. I've also replaced June's crème fraîche with yoghurt to reduce the fat.

225 g	Chana dal, soaked overnight in twice their volume of water	8 oz
50 g	Butter	1½ oz
1 tbsp	Coriander seeds	1 tbsp
1 tbsp	Cumin seeds	1 tbsp
6	Garlic cloves, peeled and finely chopped	6
2	Small red chillies, halved, de-seeded and finely chopped	2
1	Organic lemon, grated zest and juice	1
15 g	Fresh coriander, leaves and stalks separated (1 small pack)	½ oz
200 g	Natural live yoghurt	7 oz
	Sea salt and freshly ground black pepper to taste	

Drain the chana dal, rinse and boil in 1½ litres/2½ pints of water until tender and squashy (about one hour).

Dry roast the coriander and cumin seeds for 2-3 minutes, then crush them in pestle and mortar.

Melt the butter over gentle heat, add the crushed spices, garlic and half the chopped chillies and cook for 5 minutes. Add the turmeric, stir and heat gently, then remove from the heat.

Drain the chana dal, drain over a bowl and reserve the cooking liquid.

Liquidise the chana dal with some of the cooking water and purée until fine and smooth.

Add the lemon zest, coriander stalks and spices with more cooking liquid and blend until smooth.

Put everything back into the pan with the remainder of the cooking water. Bring to the boil, turn down the heat and simmer for about 30 minutes, stirring from time to time. Season to taste.

When ready to serve, add half the yoghurt and the lemon juice. Serve the soup in hot bowls with the rest of the yoghurt swirled in and scatter with the remainder of the chopped chillies and the coriander leaves.

Serves 5   **Time taken: 1¾ hours**

Per serving
Calories 245kcals; Protein 9g; Carbohydrates 30g; Sugar – Total 2g; Dietary Fibre 8g; Fat – Total 11g; Saturated Fat 5g; Vitamin C 47mg; Magnesium 62mg

I was first alerted to the nutritional benefits of chana dal by David Mendosa. David, who is a health journalist and a diabetic himself, operates a website at www.mendosa.com which is the most valuable resource for people with diabetes. Because chana dal has such a low GI (11), David devotes a whole section of his website to recipes using chana dal. Chana dal can be obtained from Asian shops and larger supermarkets and is not to be confused with split peas, which have a higher GI.

TWO-LENTIL SOUP WITH CORIANDER

Protein 21%   GI: low
Carbohydrate 61%   GL: low
Fat 18%

This is a lovely, comforting winter soup and has an interesting texture because the Puy lentils are left whole while the red lentils and vegetables are puréed. It's a good idea to make double quantities and freeze some to have on hand when you don't feel like making soup.

60 g	Puy lentils	2 oz
90 g	Split red lentils	3 oz
2 tbsp	Extra virgin olive oil	2 tbsp
1	Large onion	1

2 sticks	Celery	2 sticks
1	Large carrot	1
1/2	Red pepper	1/2
2	Garlic cloves	2
850 ml	Vegetable stock (see page 158)	1½ pints
1	Bay leaf	1
1	Organic lemon, grated zest and juice	1
1 tbsp	Concentrated tomato purée	1 tbsp
1	Bunch fresh coriander	1
	Sea salt and freshly ground black pepper	

Wash the lentils. Put the Puy lentils in a saucepan, cover with cold water, bring to the boil and cook for 30 minutes until tender. Drain well and set aside.

Meanwhile, roughly chop the onion, celery, carrot, red pepper and garlic. Gently heat the olive oil in a large saucepan, and sauté the chopped vegetables in the oil, covered, for about 10 minutes over a low heat. Add the stock, bay leaf, lemon zest (keep the juice aside for later), tomato purée and red lentils, bring to the boil and simmer over low heat for 35-40 minutes or until the vegetables are tender and the lentils have disintegrated. Remove the bay leaf and cool a little.

Wash the bunch of coriander, cutting off most of the stalks, and reserve four of the best leaves for garnish. Roughly chop the coriander and add to the cooled soup, then liquidise in a blender. If you prefer a smooth texture, rub through a sieve into a clean pan. Otherwise, return to the pan without sieving. Add the lemon juice, tasting to make sure you don't overdo it, and season to taste. Stir in the cooked Puy lentils, and reheat the soup gently. Serve in heated bowls, each serving topped with a coriander leaf.

Serves 4   **Time taken: 1 hour**

Per serving
Calories 224kcal; Protein 12g; Carbohydrates 36g; Sugar – Total 10g; Dietary Fibre 11g; Fat – Total 5g; Saturated Fat 1g; Vitamin C 67mg; Magnesium 55mg

There are lots of good reasons to increase our intake of lentils. They are a very good source of complex carbohydrates and protein, they contain a good level of B vitamins, and may help reduce 'bad' cholesterol.

ROASTED FENNEL AND RED PEPPERS WITH TAPENADE

Protein 9%
Carbohydrate 23%
Fat 68%

GI: low
GL: low

Strong colours and strong flavours make this a good dish to eat out of doors in the summer, perhaps with a glass of wine. Tapenade is a delicious olive paste sold in small jars.

2	Large red peppers	2
2	Fennel bulbs	2
2 tbsp	Extra virgin olive oil	2 tbsp
1 tbsp	Lemon juice	1 tbsp
	Sea salt and freshly ground black pepper	
4 tbsp	Tapenade	4 tbsp
2 tbsp	Pine nuts	2 tbsp
	Torn fresh basil, for garnish	

Preheat the oven to 200°C/400°F/Gas Mark 6.

Quarter the peppers and take out the seeds, then cut the quarters in half lengthways. Trim the fennel and cut downwards into quarters, then slice these in half, so that each piece is still attached at the root end. You should now have 16 pieces of each vegetable.

Place the pepper and fennel pieces on an oiled baking tray and sprinkle with the olive oil, lemon juice and seasoning. Bake the vegetables for 25-30 minutes, or until beginning to char slightly. Meanwhile, toast the pine nuts in a dry pan in the oven for no more than 5 minutes, stirring once or twice so that they are evenly browned.

To serve, place a spoonful of tapenade in the centre of each of four individual serving plates. Arrange the fennel and peppers around the tapenade like the spokes of a wheel. Sprinkle with pine nuts and torn basil leaves, and serve hot or at room temperature.

Serves 4   **Time taken: 40 minutes**

Per serving
Calories 288kcals; Protein 7g; Carbohydrates 17g; Dietary Fibre 7g; Sugar – Total 2g; Fat – Total 23g; Saturated Fat 4g; Vitamin C 86mg; Magnesium 41mg

Both peppers and fennel are said to stimulate the appetite, so that's a good enough reason to have them as a starter. Red peppers are also a rich source of vitamin C and bioflavonoids.

CHILLI MUSSELS WITH GARLIC RYE TOAST

Protein 32%
Carbohydrate 31%
Fat 37%

GI: low
GL: low

This is a twist on the classic Moules Marinières. *The addition of rye toast gives this dish an almost perfect nutritional balance.*

2.5 kg	Mussels (de-bearded and rinsed in cold water)	5 lb
2 tbsp	Extra virgin olive oil	2 tbsp
3 tbsp	White wine	3 tbsp
3	Shallots, finely chopped	3
	Freshly ground black pepper	
1	Red chilli, chopped finely	1
1	Garlic clove, crushed	1
3 tbsp	Soya cream	3 tbsp
2 tbsp	Fresh parsley, chopped	2 tbsp
	For the garlic rye toast:	
4	Slices dark rye bread or pumpernickel	4
1	Garlic clove	1
	Extra virgin olive oil, for drizzling	

Put the cleaned mussels, olive oil, white wine, shallots, seasoning, chilli and garlic into a large pan with a close-fitting lid. Put on a high heat. Once the liquid comes to the boil and the mussels start to open, add the soya cream. Continue to steam until the shells have all opened. Discard any that do not open.

For the garlic rye toast, toast the slices of rye bread, then rub with the raw garlic clove on both sides and drizzle with a few drops of olive oil.

Serve the mussels and any liquid in hot deep bowls and sprinkle generously with chopped parsley. Pass the garlic rye toast separately.

Serves 4   **Time taken: 15 minutes**

Per serving
Calories 340kcal; Protein 27g; Carbohydrates 25g; Sugar – Total 7g; Dietary Fibre 2g; Fat – Total 13g; Saturated Fat 2g; Vitamin C 45mg; Magnesium 53mg

GRILLED SARDINES WITH VEGETABLE LINGUINE

Protein 20%
Carbohydrate 27%
Fat 53%

GI: medium
GL: low

8	Fresh sardines	8
1 tbsp	Extra virgin olive oil, plus extra for brushing	1 tbsp
	Sea salt and freshly ground black pepper	
2	Medium courgettes	2
2	Medium carrots	2
2	Tomatoes, peeled, deseeded and cut into small dice	2
2	Shallots, finely chopped	2
	To serve: fresh basil leaves	

Cut off the heads of the sardines. Cut along their stomachs and open out flat. Remove any innards and the backbones. Alternatively you could ask the fishmonger to do this for you. Lay the flattened sardines on a baking tray and brush each with olive oil. Season lightly.

To make the linguine, cut the courgettes and carrots in long ribbons on a mandolin, or use a sharp knife to cut them in long slices approximately 3 mm/1/8 inch thick.

Heat the tablespoon of olive oil in a large saucepan, add the chopped shallots and cook for 3-4 minutes, without allowing them to colour, until beginning to soften.

While cooking the shallots, blanch the vegetable linguine for 15 seconds in a large pan of rapidly boiling water, then drain in a colander and add to the saucepan with the shallots. Fry on a high heat for 1 minute, then season with salt and pepper. Add the diced tomatoes. Keep warm while you grill the sardines. Preheat the grill to very hot and grill the sardines for 2-5 minutes until crisp.

Finally, spoon the courgette and carrot linguine onto individual plates, placing the sardine fillets on top, and trickle with any juices. Garnish with basil leaves.

Serves 4   Time taken: 35 minutes

Per serving
Calories 135kcal; Protein 7g; Carbohydrates 9g; Sugar – Total 4g; Dietary Fibre 3g; Fat – Total 8g; Saturated Fat 1g; Vitamin C 17mg; Magnesium 33mg

It is sometimes difficult to find our way through the plethora of food scares in the press these days. Fish are said to be full of toxins yet at the same time we are being urged to eat oily fish because they are good for our health. What should we do? Toxins become more concentrated the higher up the food chain you go, so that the carnivorous fish such as tuna and swordfish are probably less safe than the smaller fish. Sardines are a good compromise – they have all the benefits of oily fish, but are lower down the food chain.

PAN FRIED SCALLOPS WITH CABBAGE AND JUNIPER

Protein 18%   GI: low
Carbohydrate 17%   GL: low
Fat 65%

The most widely available scallops are the large king scallops, which I have used here. If, however, you are using queenies, which are smaller and cheaper, allow 5-6 per person. The coral, which is the orange part of the scallop, can be used if you like it, as I do. Some people prefer to discard it as it has quite a strong taste.

30 g	Butter	1 oz
1	Medium onion, chopped	1
1	Garlic clove, crushed	1
6	Juniper berries, lightly crushed	6
340 g	Savoy or other dark green cabbage, finely shredded	12 oz
	For the scallops:	
8-12	Large whole scallops, with coral if liked	8-12
2 tbsp	Extra virgin olive oil	2 tbsp
	Sea salt and freshly ground black pepper	

First, prepare the cabbage: melt the butter in a large saucepan. Add the onion, garlic and juniper berries and lightly cook for 5 minutes, until the onion is soft. Add the cabbage and stir until well coated with butter. Cover and cook the cabbage in its own juices for 6-7 minutes, stirring occasionally. The cabbage should be slightly crunchy and not soft.

To prepare the scallops, carefully pull the orange coral away from the ivory meat and discard the black or brown thread and the tough ligament. If the scallops are very large, slice them in half horizontally. To cook the scallops, heat the oil in a small frying pan. Pan-fry the scallops for 1-2 minutes on each side until cooked through and golden. Season to taste.

Serve the scallops on a bed of juniper cabbage.

Serves 4   **Time taken: 20 minutes**

Per serving
Calories 192kcal; Protein 9g; Carbohydrates 8g; Sugar – Total 3g; Dietary Fibre 3g; Fat – Total 14g; Saturated Fat 5g; Vitamin C 23mg; Magnesium 12mg

Juniper is a fragrant spice used to make gin. Juniper berries are good for the digestion and have antiseptic qualities as they contain a powerful antibacterial essential oil. They are also recommended for diabetes because they stimulate the pancreas.

BEANS AND GRAINS

CHILLI TOFU AND COCONUT STEW

Protein 16%
Carbohydrate 26%
Fat 58%

GI: low
GL: low

Tofu, being a curd made from soya beans, has its place here in the beans chapter. This recipe is a good introduction to tofu as it contains a variety of tastes and textures in which no single ingredient dominates, though the amount of chilli might be too strong for some palates. If you do not like hot food, seek out mild chillis and only use one.

	For the coconut broth:	
600 ml	Coconut milk	1 pint
600 ml	Vegetable stock (see page 158)	1 pint
1	Lime, grated rind only	1
450 g	Sweet potato, peeled and sliced	1 lb
450 g	Bok choy, sliced	1 lb
	For the tofu:	
2	Red chillies, seeded and chopped	2
3 tbsp	Shoyu sauce	3 tbsp
1 tbsp	Grated root ginger	1 tbsp
1 tbsp	Concentrated apple juice	1 tbsp
2 tbsp	Lime juice	2 tbsp
2 pkts	Tofu, drained, pressed and cut into small cubes (500 g/1 lb 2 oz)	2 pkts
3 tbsp	Thai basil leaves, or ordinary basil leaves, torn	3 tbsp

To make the coconut broth, put the coconut milk, vegetable stock and grated lime rind in a large pan over medium heat. Add the sweet potato and cook, covered, for 10 minutes. Add the bok choy and cook for a further 4-5 minutes, or until the vegetables are tender. Keep warm.

Cook the tofu at the same time. Place the chillies, Shoyu, ginger, concentrated apple juice and lime juice in a frying pan over medium heat and cook for 3 minutes. Add the cubed tofu to the pan and cook for one minute on each side or until coated with the chilli sauce.

To serve, spoon the coconut broth, sweet potato and bok choy into deep bowls. Top with the chilli tofu and sprinkle with basil leaves.

Serves 6   **Time taken: 20 minutes**

Per serving
Calories 391kcal; Protein 17g; Carbohydrates 26g; Sugar – Total 14g; Dietary Fibre 4g; Fat – Total 26g; Saturated Fat 19g; Vitamin C 70mg; Magnesium 84mg

There are various kinds of soy sauce on the market. The only two I use are Shoyu and Tamari, both of which are naturally brewed. Shoyu contains wheat and is a little lighter; it also stands up better to cooking than Tamari, which has a stronger taste. I use Tamari at the end of a dish as a condiment rather than as a cooking ingredient. Avoid commercial soy sauces altogether – these often have added salt or monosodium glutamate.

TOFU FAJITAS

Protein 20%   GI: medium
Carbohydrate 30%   GL: medium
Fat 50%

You can buy ready-made flour tortillas, but make sure they are made from whole wheat flour and not refined white flour. If you can't find ready-made ones, it's not difficult to make your own, just a bit time-consuming.

	For the tortillas:	
110 g	Organic wholemeal flour	4 oz
	Pinch of sea salt	
2 tbsp	Extra virgin olive oil	2 tbsp
5 tbsp	Warm water	5 tbsp
	For the filling:	
2 tbsp	Extra virgin olive oil	2 tbsp
1	Large onion, sliced	1
1	Red pepper, seeded and sliced thinly	1

1	Green pepper, seeded and sliced thinly	1
1	Hot chilli pepper, seeded and finely diced	1
110 g	Mushrooms, sliced	4 oz
450 g	Tofu (2 packets), drained and pressed to extract excess moisture	1 lb
	Sea salt	
	Any of the following as a garnish:	
	Natural live yoghurt	
	Chopped fresh coriander	
	Chopped fresh tomatoes	
	Sliced avocado	
	Spring onions	

For the tortillas, combine the flour and salt in a bowl. Add the oil, and gradually add enough water to make a soft dough. Divide the dough into 6 pieces. Shape each piece into a small, smooth ball. Flatten the balls with a rolling pin, and roll each one out on a lightly floured surface to a circle about 17.5 cm/7 inches in diameter. Roll out no more than two at a time to prevent their drying out. Cook in an ungreased heavy frying pan or direct on a hot griddle until the top is bubbled and the underside flecked with brown. Turn it over and cook the other side. Stack the cooked tortillas in a warm place and cover with a cloth.

Heat the olive oil in a large frying pan over medium-high heat, then add the onions. Sauté, stirring, until the onions are translucent. Stir in the peppers and mushrooms and sauté until the vegetables begin to soften, about 5 minutes. Add the tofu and stir-fry for 5 minutes more. Season with salt to taste and serve in the tortillas.

Serve the fajitas with yoghurt, chopped coriander, chopped fresh tomatoes, avocado, spring onions, or a combination of these.

Serves 6   **Time taken: 1 hour**

Per serving (without garnish)
Calories 383kcals; Protein 20g; Carbohydrates 30g; Dietary Fibre 6g; Sugar – Total 5g; Fat – Total 22g; Saturated Fat 4g; Vitamin C 113mg; Magnesium 85mg

A number of studies have confirmed that 25-50 g soya protein, such as that found in tofu, eaten daily for four weeks, can decrease LDL, the 'bad' cholesterol, by as much as 10-20% in people with raised blood cholesterol.

SOYA BEAN AND
MANGO CHUTNEY CASSEROLE

Protein 14%

GI: low

Carbohydrate 38%

GL: low

Fat 48%

This is an adaptation of the very first vegetarian dish I ever cooked, from Anna Thomas's The Vegetarian Epicure, *which was published in the UK in 1973, and was an inspiration to a whole generation of vegetarian cooks.*

225 g	Dried soya beans, soaked overnight	8 oz
1	Thumb-sized piece of root ginger, peeled	1
3 tbsp	Mango chutney, large pieces of mango chopped finely	3 tbsp
1	400g tin chopped Italian tomatoes	1
1½ tsp	Dried mustard powder	1½ tsp
3 tbsp	Extra virgin olive oil	3 tbsp
3	Medium onions, peeled and chopped	3
3 tbsp	Blackstrap molasses	3 tbsp

Drain and rinse the soya beans, then place in a large saucepan and cover with cold water. Add the ginger. Bring to the boil, reduce the heat, cover and cook until tender – this can take as long as 3 hours, even longer than chickpeas. Check the liquid level every now and again, and add water as necessary. Drain, reserving 300 ml/½ pint of the cooking liquid.

Meanwhile, heat the olive oil in a large frying pan, and cook the chopped onions until golden.

Put everything into a large casserole – soaked beans, chutney, tomatoes and their juice, mustard powder, cooked onions and molasses and the reserved bean liquor. Cover and bake for 1-1½ hours until the beans are tender and the liquid thickened.

Serves 4   **Time taken: 4½ hours plus soaking**

Per serving
Calories 314kcal; Protein 12g; Carbohydrates 31g; Sugar – Total 15g; Dietary Fibre 5g; Fat – Total 17g; Saturated Fat 2g; Vitamin C 15mg; Magnesium 93mg

At 18, soya beans have one of the lowest GI values so far measured. In traditional Chinese medicine soya beans are believed to have 'cooling' properties that cleanse the blood and, crucially for people with diabetes, strengthen the pancreas. They are rich in potassium, and may be helpful in controlling high blood pressure.

BUTTER BEANS WITH FENNEL

Protein 17%   GI: low
Carbohydrate 56%   GL: low
Fat 27%

I've come quite late to butter beans, having been force-fed them as a child, but now regard them as one of my favourite beans. They must be cooked well, until they melt in the mouth but still hold their shape. This dish could be served as an accompaniment to fish or chicken, or as a light meal in its own right.

300 g	Butter beans, soaked overnight	10 oz
1	Thumb-sized piece of ginger root, peeled	1
3 tbsp	Extra virgin olive oil	3 tbsp
2 tbsp	Fennel seeds	2 tbsp
3	Garlic cloves, chopped	3
2	Large onions, cut into wedges	2
2	Fennel roots, trimmed and cut into wedges through the root	2
1	Lemon, juice only	1
	Sea salt and freshly ground black pepper	
2 tbsp	Fresh parsley, chopped	2 tbsp
1 tbsp	Fresh chives, chopped	1 tbsp
1 tbsp	Fresh dill, chopped	1 tbsp

Drain the butter beans of their soaking water and put in a large pan with cold water to cover. Add the ginger. Bring to the boil, reduce the heat, cover and cook for 1-1½ hours, or until tender. Drain, reserving 425 ml/¾ pint of the cooking liquid.

Heat 2 tablespoons of the olive oil in a large pan over gentle heat. Add the fennel seeds, garlic and onions, and sauté for 5-10 minutes until softened. Add the fennel together with the reserved cooking liquid, and cook for 10-15 minutes, until the fennel is tender but still has some 'bite'. There should still be a little liquid left.

Add the drained beans, the remainder of the olive oil, lemon juice and seasoning. Reheat until piping hot and serve sprinkled liberally with the fresh herbs.

Serves 6   **Time taken: 2 hours**

Per serving
Calories 254kcals; Protein 11g; Carbohydrates 37g; Dietary Fibre 12g; Sugar – Total 7g; Fat – Total 8g; Saturated Fat 1g; Vitamin C 16mg; Magnesium 74mg

Butter beans are believed to neutralise acidity in the stomach that arises from a meat-rich diet. Like all beans, they have cholesterol-lowering and blood pressure-lowering properties as well, probably as a result of the protein and fibre they contain.

CHANA DAL WITH SPINACH

Protein 21%   GI: very low
Carbohydrate 53%   GL: very low
Fat 26%

This recipe comes from Jane Sen, who is the Dietary Advisor to the Bristol Cancer Help Centre, where I have attended a course in nutrition for cancer. Jane uses yellow split peas, but the substitution of chana dal makes this dish very low GI and therefore even more suitable for people with diabetes.

225 g	Chana dal, washed and soaked overnight	8 oz
1.2 litres	Vegetable stock (see page 158)	2 pints
1 tsp	Turmeric	1 tsp
2 tbsp	Extra virgin olive oil	2 tbsp
2	Bay leaves	2
1 tsp	Black mustard seeds	1 tsp
1 tsp	Cumin seeds	1 tsp
1	Cinnamon stick	1
4	Whole cloves	4
2.5 cm	Fresh ginger root, peeled and grated	1 inch
350 g	Spinach leaves, washed and roughly chopped	12 oz

Drain the chana dal. Put it in a large pan with the stock. Bring to the boil over medium heat. Add the turmeric. Reduce the heat and simmer, covered, for an hour until the dal is tender. Remove from the heat.

Heat the oil in a large pan, add the bay leaves, mustard seeds, cumin seeds, cinnamon and cloves and cook until the spices release their aroma. Add the grated ginger and chopped spinach. Stir to coat with the oil and spices. When the spinach has wilted, stir in the chana dal. Reduce the heat and cook for 3 minutes or so, then serve hot with brown basmati rice.

Serves 4   **Time taken: 1¼ hours**

Per serving
Calories 295kcals; Protein 16g; Carbohydrates 40g; Dietary Fibre 16g; Sugar – Total 8g; Fat – Total 9g; Saturated Fat 1g; Vitamin C 15mg; Magnesium 121mg

LENTIL AND SWEET POTATO CURRY WITH BROCCOLI

Protein 21%   GI: medium
Carbohydrate 53%   GL: low
Fat 26%

Use the green or brown continental lentils for this dish, or Puy lentils. The red lentils disintegrate on cooking whereas you want the lentils to stay intact. This curry is quite substantial – more of a main meal than a side dish.

100g	Green or brown lentils	3½ oz
2 tbsp	Extra virgin olive oil	2 tbsp
1	Onion, peeled and thinly sliced	1
2	Garlic cloves, peeled and finely chopped	2
2.5 cm	Fresh ginger root, peeled and finely chopped	1 inch
½	Fresh green chilli, seeded and finely chopped	½
1 tsp	Cumin seeds	1 tsp
1 tsp	Coriander seeds, lightly crushed	1 tsp
½ tsp	Turmeric	½ tsp
2	Sweet potatoes, peeled and cut into chunks	2
	Sea salt to taste	

2	400g cans chopped tomatoes	2
200 g	Broccoli, broken into small florets and lightly steamed	7 oz

Wash the lentils, put them in a pan and cover with cold water. Bring to the boil, reduce the heat and simmer until tender – about 20 minutes. Drain and reserve.

Heat the oil in a large pan, and sauté the onion, garlic, ginger and chilli over a low heat until softened but not browned – 5-8 minutes. Add the spices and cook for another 3 minutes or so, stirring from time to time, until the spices release their aroma. Add the sweet potatoes and a little sea salt, and stir. Then add the chopped tomatoes and their juice, bring to the boil, cover and simmer for 20 minutes, or until the sweet potato is nearly tender. Now add the reserved cooked lentils and cook for another 5 minutes. Stir in the steamed broccoli florets, cover again and leave on a low heat for another couple of minutes until the broccoli has warmed through. Stir well and serve hot.

Serves 4   **Time taken: 1 hour**

Per serving
Calories 305kcals; Protein 13g; Carbohydrates 50g; Dietary Fibre 14g; Sugar – Total 10g; Fat – Total 8g; Saturated Fat 1g; Vitamin C 89mg; Magnesium 101mg

Lentils are a valuable food for people with diabetes because they contain both soluble and insoluble fibre when helps to stabilise blood glucose levels and lower raised blood fats. Their GI is low at 29-30.

PUY LENTILS WITH OLIVES AND ANCHOVIES

Protein 20%   GI: low
Carbohydrate 38%   GL: low
Fat 42%

Puy lentils are everybody's favourite lentil, which is probably why most of the world's supply comes, not from the Le Puy region of France any more, but from Canada, which is able to produce them in larger quantities. They have a wonderful earthy taste, and go well with the strong flavours of olives and anchovies – truly a taste of the warm South. This dish can be served hot or at room temperature, and is even better the next day.

350 g	Puy lentils	12 oz
2	Garlic cloves, peeled	2
2	2 oz tins of anchovies, drained and rinsed	2
6 tbsp	Extra virgin olive oil	6 tbsp
1/2	Lemon, juice only	1/2
	Freshly ground black pepper	
18-24	Black olives, preferably Kalamata	18-24
2 tbsp	Fresh flat leaf parsley, chopped	2 tbsp
2 tbsp	Fresh coriander, chopped	2 tbsp

Wash the lentils and put in a pan with cold water to cover. Bring to the boil and cook for about 20 minutes until tender but still retaining their shape.

Put the garlic and half the anchovies in the blender with the olive oil and blend to a smooth purée. Chop the remaining anchovies and tip into a small saucepan together with the garlic and anchovy purée. Heat gently.

When the lentils are cooked, drain and put in a serving bowl. Add the anchovy mixture and toss well. Add the lemon juice and pepper and taste – you may require more lemon juice. Mix in the olives and chopped parsley and coriander, and serve hot.

Serves 4 **Time taken: 30 minutes**

Per serving
Calories 566kcals; Protein 27g; Carbohydrates 54g; Dietary Fibre 13g; Sugar – Total 4g; Fat – Total 27g; Saturated Fat 3g; Vitamin C 6mg; Magnesium 17mg

Both lentils and anchovies are very good sources of iron. Anchovies contain more protein, gram for gram, than any other oily fish, together with loads of calcium and vitamin B12. This is important as vitamin B12 is needed for the production of red blood cells and DNA and is involved in maintaining the health of the nervous system.

SCOTCH EGGS WITH A DIFFERENCE

Protein 19%
Carbohydrate 38%
Fat 43%

GI: low
GL: low

I always loved Scotch Eggs as a child – looking back now I shudder to think of the amount of saturated fat they contained. These are much more nutritious and not as time consuming as you might think, especially if you use tinned chickpeas.

2	400 g cans of chickpeas (or use 200 g/7 oz dried chickpeas, soaked and cooked until tender)	2
2	Garlic cloves, crushed	2
1	Fresh red chilli, deseeded and finely chopped	1
2	Plum tomatoes, skinned, deseeded and finely chopped	2
4	Spring onions, chopped	4
110 g	Black olives, stoned and chopped	4 oz
4 tbsp	Flat leaf parsley, chopped	4 tbsp
	Sea salt and freshly ground black pepper	
6	Organic free range eggs, hard-boiled	6
1	Organic free range egg, beaten	1
4 tbsp	Dry polenta	4 tbsp
2 tbsp	Extra virgin olive oil	2 tbsp

Preheat the oven to 200°C/400°F/Gas Mark 6.

If using canned chickpeas, drain and rinse them. Place the chickpeas in the food processor with the garlic and process until chopped. Turn out into a bowl and add the chillies, tomatoes, spring onions, olives and parsley. Season to taste and mix well.

Divide the mixture into six equal portions, and flatten out. Now, using your hands, press the mixture onto the outsides of the six hard-boiled eggs so that each egg is completely encased. Make sure that the surface of the eggs is dry.

Next, dip the coated eggs in beaten egg and then in polenta and place on an oiled baking sheet.

Spray the Scotch eggs the with olive oil spray or drizzle with a little olive oil, and bake in the preheated oven for 20-30 minutes, or until golden, turning once. Serve with a green salad.

Serves 6   **Time taken: 1 hour**

Per serving
Calories 309kcals; Protein 15g; Carbohydrates 30g; Dietary Fibre 7g; Sugar – Total 3g; Fat – Total 15g; Saturated Fat 3g; Vitamin C 30mg; Magnesium 47mg

This recipe has a good nutritional profile – lots of protein and minerals in the eggs and chickpeas. Among other nutrients, eggs contain selenium and vitamin E, both known to have antioxidant properties that may reduce the risk of damage to blood vessel walls and therefore the likelihood of heart disease developing. This is particularly important for people with diabetes as their heart disease risk is elevated.

GRAINS

By their very nature, grains are high in carbohydrate, so it's very difficult to make a grain-based dish yield much less than 50 g of carbohydrate per serving. However, I have used low GI grains such as pearl barley, brown rice and polenta; or foods which are not grains at all, though they cook like grains and are commonly classified as such. These are quinoa, amaranth, wild rice and buckwheat. Buckwheat in particular has the added advantage of actually increasing insulin sensitivity in people with diabetes. Therefore none of the recipes that follow should have an undue effect on blood glucose. Most of the recipes are designed as light meals for 4 people, but could stretch to feeding 6 people as a side dish.

CRISPY POLENTA WITH WILD MUSHROOMS AND CORIANDER PESTO

Protein 8%
Carbohydrate 13%
Fat 79%

GI: medium
GL: medium

I think that this is absolutely the best way to serve polenta. Don't worry if you can't find wild mushrooms. You can use chestnut mushrooms instead, or even ordinary white ones. If you use dried wild mushrooms, reconstitute them in hot water as directed on the packet, then use the soaking water instead of vegetable stock.

200 g	Instant polenta	7 oz
2 tbsp	Extra virgin olive oil	2 tbsp
225 g	Mixed wild mushrooms, cleaned and sliced	8 oz
1 tsp	Chopped fresh rosemary	1 tsp
2 tsp	Chopped fresh thyme	2 tsp
2	Garlic cloves, peeled and crushed	2
	Freshly ground black pepper	
150 ml	Vegetable stock (see page 158)	1/4 pint
3 tbsp	Soya cream	3 tbsp
	For the coriander pesto:	
large handful	Packed fresh coriander leaves	large handful
6 tbsp	Extra virgin olive oil	6 tbsp
1	Garlic clove	1
100 g	Pine nuts, almonds or cashews	3 1/2 oz
2 tbsp	Lemon juice	2 tbsp

Bring 725 ml/1¼ pints of water to boil in a medium saucepan. Pour in the polenta gradually, stirring with a wooden spoon as you do so. Reduce the heat to medium, and cook, stirring constantly, for 5 minutes, until thick. Oil a 25 x 30 cm/10 x 12 inch baking sheet, then pour in the cooked polenta so that it makes a layer about 5 mm/¼ inch thick. Leave to cool completely.

When the polenta is cold, cut it into 12 squares or circles about 8 cm/3 inches in diameter. Place in a very low oven – 70°C/150°F/ Gas Mark ¼ – and leave for several hours or overnight to dry out completely. It should become quite crisp.

For the mushrooms, heat the olive oil in a wok or large pan, add the mushrooms, rosemary, thyme, garlic and seasoning, and stir fry for 3-4 minutes. Pour in the stock and continue cooking until the stock has reduced by half. Stir in the soya cream and simmer for another 3-4 minutes until thick and creamy.

For the coriander pesto, put the coriander and olive oil in a blender and process until the coriander is finely chopped. Add the rest of the ingredients and process until you have a lumpy paste (you may have to add a little hot water and scrape down the sides of the blender). This can be done in advance.

To assemble the dish, warm the polenta slices, then spread them with coriander pesto. Layer on individual plates with the mushroom mixture and serve warm.

Serves 4   **Time taken: 20 minutes plus cooling and drying**

Per serving
Calories 406kcals; Protein 7g; Carbohydrates 14g; Dietary Fibre 3g; Sugar – Total 2g; Fat – Total 37g; Saturated Fat 5g; Vitamin C 8mg; Magnesium 52mg

The recipe for coriander pesto comes from Karen Watkins of Mineral Check, a company that analyses hair samples for toxic minerals and trace minerals. Coriander contains selenium and selenium opposes mercury, so Karen recommends that anyone who is found to have high mercury should eat two tablespoons a day of this delicious pesto.

BARLEY AND SPRING VEGETABLE RISOTTO

Protein 16%   GI: low
Carbohydrate 59%   GL: low
Fat 25%

I have used Parmesan in this risotto, because it does enhance the flavour. If, however, you are avoiding all dairy products, toasted sesame or sunflower seeds make a good and tasty alternative.

2 tbsp	Extra virgin olive oil	2 tbsp
1	Large onion, peeled and finely chopped	1
1	Garlic clove, finely chopped	1
300 g	Pearl barley	10½ oz
150 ml	White wine	¼ pint
600 ml	Vegetable stock (see page 158)	1 pint
100 g	Peas, fresh or frozen	3½ oz
2	Small courgettes, thinly sliced	2
1	Bunch of asparagus, trimmed and chopped into 1 cm/½ inch lengths (set aside the asparagus tips)	1
2	Medium tomatoes, peeled, deseeded and chopped	2
3 tbsp	Mint leaves, finely chopped	3 tbsp
2 tbsp	Parsley, finely chopped	2 tbsp
2 tbsp	Parmesan cheese, finely grated	2 tbsp
	Sea salt and freshly ground black pepper	
	To serve:	
1 tbsp	Parmesan, shaved	1 tbsp
4 tbsp	Pine nuts, lightly toasted	4 tbsp
	Asparagus tips (reserved) blanched in boiling water for 1 minute	
1 tbsp	Fresh basil leaves, torn	1 tbsp

Place the olive oil in a large saucepan over a moderate heat. When the oil is hot add the onion and cook until transparent. Add the garlic and barley to the pan and cook, stirring frequently, for 2-3 minutes. Add the white wine and continue to cook and stir until the wine has evaporated.

Meanwhile bring the stock to the boil in a separate saucepan.

Gradually stir a cupful of boiling stock into the barley mixture. Bring the stock to a steady simmer and cook for 50 minutes stirring it regularly, adding the hot stock cupful by cupful until almost all of it has been absorbed. By this time the barley should be tender with a little bite to it. If it is still firm add a little more stock or water and allow it to cook for a further 5-10 minutes.

Stir in the peas, sliced courgettes and chopped asparagus and cook them with the barley for 5-8 minutes until the vegetables are tender.

Remove the risotto from the heat and stir in the mint, parsley, tomatoes, seasoning and Parmesan, and mix it until well distributed.

To serve, spoon the risotto into heated serving bowls and garnish with the reserved asparagus tips, pine nuts, basil and Parmesan shavings.

Serves 6   **Time taken: 1¼ hours**

Per serving
Calories 347kcals; Protein 12g; Carbohydrates 54g; Dietary Fibre 12g; Sugar – Total 8g; Fat – Total 9g; Saturated Fat 2g; Vitamin C 26mg; Magnesium 85mg

Pearl barley is not a whole grain, as the husk has been removed. However, it is extremely useful for people with diabetes as it has a low GI – at 25, it is the lowest of all grains.

QUINOA PILAFF WITH GREEN LEAVES

Protein 11%   GI: medium
Carbohydrate 58%   GL: medium
Fat 31%

If you can't find quinoa, you could substitute pearl barley in this pilaff, but it would need considerably more cooking time – about 1¼ hours.

225 g	Quinoa	8 oz
600 ml	Vegetable stock (see page 158)	1 pint
3 tbsp	Extra virgin olive oil	3 tbsp
4 tsp	Cumin seeds	4 tsp
1	Cinnamon stick	1
1	Onion, peeled and finely chopped	1
450 g	Green leaves, such as Swiss chard,	1 lb

	beetroot leaves, spring greens, spinach or dark green cabbage leaves, finely shredded	
4 tbsp	Raisins	4 tbsp
	Sea salt and freshly ground black pepper	
1	Lemon, finely grated rind and juice	1
1	Large carrot, peeled if not organic, and grated	1
2 tbsp	Fresh coriander, chopped	2 tbsp

Wash the quinoa well as it is coated with a natural substance called saponin, which may taste bitter. Drain thoroughly, then put in a saucepan with the stock. Bring to the boil, lower the heat, cover and simmer for 15 minutes until nearly tender and most of the liquid is absorbed.

Meanwhile, heat the olive oil in a pan over medium heat and add the chopped onion, cumin seeds and cinnamon stick. Sauté gently for 5-8 minutes until the onion is soft but not browned. Add the onion, spices and oil to the simmering quinoa and stir.

Add the shredded green leaves, raisins, seasoning and lemon rind and juice to the pan, cover tightly and continue cooking for another 5 minutes. When the quinoa is tender and there is no liquid left, stir in the grated carrot, adjust the seasoning, and serve sprinkled with chopped coriander.

Serves 4   **Time taken: 30 minutes**

Per serving
Calories 412kcals; Protein 11g; Carbohydrates 62g; Dietary Fibre 8g; Sugar – Total 13g; Fat – Total 15g; Saturated Fat 2g; Vitamin C 29mg; Magnesium 226mg

Quinoa is not officially a grain at all, but a seed. It is extremely high in fibre, low in fat and very high in protein. It contains the correct balance of amino acids. The combination of quinoa and greens makes this recipe the richest source of magnesium in the book.

AMARANTH AND LENTIL CAKES

Protein 13%　　　　　　　　　　　　　　　　GI: medium
Carbohydrate 45%　　　　　　　　　　　　　GL: medium
Fat 42%

This dish is based loosely on a traditional Armenian recipe, though traditionally bulgur wheat would have been used rather than amaranth. The cakes go well with a fresh tomato sauce such as that on page 161.

110 g	Red lentils	4 oz
425 ml	Water	15 fl oz
90 g	Amaranth	3 oz
4 tbsp	Extra virgin olive oil	4 tbsp
1	Medium onion, peeled and finely chopped	1
1/2	Red pepper, seeded and finely chopped	1/2
1/2	Green pepper, seeded and finely chopped	1/2
6	Spring onions, finely chopped	6
2 tbsp	Fresh flat leaf parsley, finely chopped	2 tbsp
1 tsp	Paprika	1 tsp
2 tbsp	Fresh mint, chopped	2 tbsp
	Sea salt and freshly ground black pepper	
	Olive oil spray for frying	

Put the lentils, amaranth and water into a large saucepan. Bring to the boil, then lower the heat and simmer for 20 minutes until the lentils and amaranth are tender. Stir in two tablespoonfuls of olive oil and set aside.

Heat the remaining olive oil in a frying pan and sauté the chopped onion for about 10 minutes, until golden, stirring frequently. In a large bowl, mix together the lentils, amaranth and onions. Add the red and green peppers, spring onions, parsley, paprika, mint and seasoning. Mix well with your hands, then form the mixture into 12 equal-sized patties.

Spray a large frying pan with olive oil spray and fry the patties over moderate heat, turning once, until golden.

Serves 4　　　　　　　　　　　　　　　Time taken: 1 hour

Per serving
Calories 327kcals; Protein 11g; Carbohydrates 37g; Dietary

Fibre 9g; Sugar – Total 4g; Fat – Total 16g; Saturated Fat 2g;
Vitamin C 49mg; Magnesium 71mg

Amaranth was a staple in the diets of pre-Columbian Aztecs,
who believed it had supernatural powers and incorporated it
into their religious ceremonies. Amaranth has a "sticky" texture
that contrasts with the fluffier texture of most grains and care
should be taken not to overcook it as it can become gummy.
Amaranth seed is high in protein (15-18%) and contains
respectable amounts of lysine and methionine, two essential
amino acids that are not frequently found in grains. It is high in
fibre and contains calcium, iron, potassium, phosphorus, and
vitamins A and C. The fibre content of amaranth is three times
that of wheat and its iron content, five times more than wheat.
It contains twice as much calcium as milk
    Amaranth also contains tocotrienols (a form of vitamin E)
which have cholesterol-lowering activity.

BUCKWHEAT WITH ROASTED AUBERGINE

Protein 12%   GI: medium
Carbohydrate 62%   GL: medium
Fat 26%

*Kasha or buckwheat comes as small triangular-shaped grains, and is
actually a member of the grass family and not a wheat at all, and
has therefore the supreme advantage of being gluten-free. You can
buy buckwheat roasted or unroasted. I usually buy the unroasted
sort, which is a greenish colour, and roast it myself. If you buy the
roasted kind, you do not need to sauté it first, but just wash it and
put in the pan with the stock, garlic and bay leaf.*

1	Large aubergine, cut in half vertically	1
1	Red pepper, deseeded and cut in half vertically	1
3 tbsp	Extra virgin olive oil	3 tbsp
225 g	Buckwheat	8 oz
2	Garlic cloves, peeled and finely chopped	2
500 ml	Vegetable stock (see page 158)	18 fl oz
1	Bay leaf	1
1	Lemon, juice only	1
1 tsp	Chopped fresh sage	1 tsp

1 tsp	Chopped fresh thyme	1 tsp
2 tbsp	Torn fresh basil leaves	2 tbsp

Preheat the oven to 200°C/400°F/Gas Mark 6.

Put the halved aubergine and pepper on a baking sheet. Sprinkle with one tablespoon of olive oil, then bake in the preheated oven for 25-30 minutes, or until just starting to char. Take out of the oven and put the vegetables into a paper bag, fold to seal and set aside.

In a large frying pan, heat the oil over medium heat. Add the buckwheat and sauté for about five minutes, until fragrant. Add the garlic, stock, and bay leaf, then cover and simmer until all the liquid is absorbed – this should take about 15 minutes.

Add the lemon juice, sage and thyme to the buckwheat and stir well.

Remove the pepper and aubergine from the bag and remove the charred skins with your fingers. Chop the vegetables, add them to the buckwheat and stir well.

Remove the bay leaf, then place the mixture in a serving dish and serve warm sprinkled liberally with the torn basil leaves.

Serves 4   **Time taken: 1 hour, 10 minutes**

Per serving
Calories 305kcals; Protein 9g; Carbohydrates 51g; Dietary Fibre 9g; Sugar – Total 7g; Fat – Total 9g; Saturated Fat 1g; Vitamin C 65mg; Magnesium 150mg

Buckwheat is one of the most beneficial grains for people with diabetes. It is not related to wheat, and is not even, technically, a grain, but a fruit. Several studies have shown that buckwheat may help increase insulin sensitivity. A component of buckwheat called chiro-inositol, which is relatively high in buckwheat but rarely found in other foods, appears to prompt cells to become more insulin-sensitive. In animal studies it has been shown to lower blood glucose levels, and it has the added benefit of containing good levels of B vitamins and omega-3 fatty acids, as well as acting as a prebiotic, encouraging the growth of 'friendly' bacteria in the digestive tract.

BUCKWHEAT NOODLES WITH TOFU, TAHINI SAUCE AND VEGETABLES

Protein 22%
Carbohydrate 53%
Fat 25%

GI: medium
GL: low

Like amaranth, buckwheat is not strictly a grain or cereal at all, but the seed of a flowering thistle. However, because its consistency and nutrient content is similar to a cereal, it is treated like one.

250 g	Tofu (1 pack)	8¹/₂ oz
1	Piece of fresh ginger root, about 2.5 cm/1 inch, peeled and grated	1
2 tbsp	Tamari	2 tbsp
1 tbsp	Rice vinegar	1 tbsp
225 g	Soba noodles (buckwheat noodles)	8 oz
1 tbsp	Extra virgin olive oil	1 tbsp
1	Medium onion, peeled and finely chopped	1
2	Carrots, peeled unless organic, and sliced thinly	2
1	Garlic clove, finely chopped	1
2	Small courgettes, sliced thinly	2
2 tbsp	Fresh coriander leaves, chopped	2 tbsp
	For the sauce:	
2 tbsp	Tahini	2 tbsp
2 tbsp	Tamari	2 tbsp

First, marinate the tofu: drain, rinse and press it dry, then cut into 1 cm/¹/₂ inch cubes and place in a bowl. Mix together the grated ginger, tamari and rice vinegar and pour over the tofu, stirring gently to coat. Leave to marinate for at least 30 minutes.

Heat the olive oil in a wide pan, and sauté the onion for 5-8 minutes until soft but not browned. Add the carrot and garlic and continue to sauté for another 3 minutes. Add the courgette and cook for another minute or two.

Finally, stir in the chopped coriander. Keep warm.

Drain the tofu and discard the marinade. Grill the tofu under a hot grill, turning once or twice, until golden.

For the sauce, mix together the tahini, tamari and 6 tablespoons of water in a small bowl.

Cook the soba noodles according to the directions on the packet

– they need considerably less time that wheat pasta – about 5-6 minutes. Be careful not to let them overcook or they can become gummy. Drain well, then return to the pan and stir in the tahini sauce, the grilled tofu cubes and the vegetables. Serve in heated bowls.

Serves 4   **Time taken: 1 hour 10 minutes**

Per serving
Calories 407kcals; Protein 23g; Carbohydrates 57g; Dietary Fibre 5g; Sugar – Total 5g; Fat – Total 12g; Saturated Fat 2g; Vitamin C 9mg; Magnesium 73mg

This is the highest protein grain dish in this section, mainly due to the combination of tofu and buckwheat. If you do not like tofu, substituting cubed skinless chicken breast would have the same effect.

BUCKWHEAT PANCAKES WITH RATATOUILLE

Protein 13%　　　　　　　　　　　　GI: low
Carbohydrate 54%　　　　　　　　　GL: medium
Fat 33%

These pancakes are extremely versatile; they can be served with a savoury accompaniment as here, or with some guacamole or salsa, or at breakfast time rolled round some poached apple and a sprinkling of cinnamon. They can be made with all buckwheat flour, but I have added a little mixed gluten-free flour to lighten the mixture.

There are almost as many versions of ratatouille as there are cooks. This is my current favourite in which the vegetables are roasted first.

	For the pancakes:	
90 g	Buckwheat flour	3 oz
30 g	Unbleached white flour or gluten-free flour	1 oz
1	Large, organic free range egg	1
1 tbsp	Flax seeds, ground finely	1 tbsp
275 ml	Soya, nut or rice milk	½ pint
	For the ratatouille:	
1	Large onion, peeled and sliced downwards, from stem to root	1

1	Medium aubergine, cut into ³/₄ inch/2 cm chunks	1
1 sprig	Fresh rosemary	1 sprig
2 tbsp	Extra virgin olive oil	2 tbsp
1	Garlic clove, peeled and chopped	1
3	Small courgettes, sliced into ¹/₂ inch slices	3
1	Red pepper, cored, deseeded and cut into ³/₄ inch/2 cm squares	1
450 g	Fresh ripe tomatoes, peeled, deseeded and chopped	1 lb
	Sea salt and freshly ground black pepper to taste	
	Torn fresh basil leaves and 4 sprigs of basil, for garnish	

First, mix the batter for the pancakes. Put all the ingredients into the blender and blend to mix, scraping down the sides of the goblet to make sure the mixture is well amalgamated. Set aside for at least half an hour, then give another whiz before using.

Meanwhile, make the ratatouille. Preheat oven to 200°C/400°F/ Gas Mark 6.

Spray a roasting pan with olive oil and place the onion and aubergine in it. Strip the rosemary leaves off their stem and add to the pan. Sprinkle a little olive oil over the vegetables, then roast for 10 minutes. Add the courgettes and peppers and roast for another 15 minutes.

Put the chopped tomatoes in a pan and add the roasted vegetables. Season to taste, then cook for 15 minutes over a low heat.

For the pancakes, heat a heavy bottomed frying pan, then oil lightly. I find my olive oil spray invaluable for this, as it uses the minimum of oil. Pour a little batter into the pan and swirl around until the bottom is entirely covered. Cook until a few bubbles appear on the surface, then flip it over and cook the other side for a couple of minutes. Stack the pancakes on a warm plate and cover with a tea towel while you make the remaining pancakes.

To serve, fold the pancakes into quarters to make a cone shape, then fill the cone with ratatouille. Serve sprinkled with torn basil leaves and a sprig of basil.

Serves 4   Time taken: 1¹/₄ hours

Per serving
Calories 304kcals; Protein 11g; Carbohydrates 44g; Dietary Fibre 8g; Sugar – Total 12g; Fat – Total 12g; Saturated Fat 2g; Vitamin C 83mg; Magnesium 129mg

POULTRY AND FISH

CHICKEN IN COCONUT MILK

Protein 60%   GI: low
Carbohydrate 8%   GL: low
Fat 32%

I always insist on organic, free range chicken. There are so many questionable practices in the poultry industry that it is worth paying the extra for good quality and peace of mind, even if it means you don't eat chicken as often as you have been used to.

4	Organic chicken breasts, skinned and sliced diagonally	4
1 tbsp	Coconut oil	1 tbsp
2.5 cm	Piece of ginger root, peeled and cut into fine julienne	1 inch
1	Fresh red chilli, seeded and finely chopped	1
1	Garlic clove, peeled and finely chopped	1
350 ml	Coconut milk	12 fl oz
350 ml	Chicken stock (see page 159)	12 fl oz
1	Large handful fresh basil, torn	1
100 g	Fresh mung bean sprouts, washed	3½ oz

Heat the coconut oil in a wok or large frying pan over medium heat. Toss in the sliced chicken and stir fry until sealed. Remove the chicken and set aside. Add the ginger, chilli, garlic, coconut milk and chicken stock and bring to the boil. Turn down the heat and simmer for 5 minutes.

Return the chicken to the pan and cook for another 5 minutes, or until the chicken has cooked through. Stir in the torn basil leaves. Put the beansprouts into heated serving bowls and spoon the chicken and coconut milk sauce over the top. Serve very hot.

Serves 4   **Time taken: 25 minutes**

Per serving
Calories 197kcals; Protein 29g; Carbohydrates 4g; Dietary Fibre 1g; Sugar – Total 1g; Fat – Total 7g; Saturated Fat 4g; Vitamin C 33mg; Magnesium 58mg

Mung bean sprouts are thought to be beneficial as an antidiabetic, low glycaemic index food, rich in antioxidants.

GRILLED CHICKEN WITH QUINOA AND LEMONS

Protein 30%
Carbohydrate 17%
Fat 53%

GI: low
GL: low

The chicken can be cooked on the barbecue or under a grill, but I always take the precaution of baking the chicken first to make sure it is cooked through to the middle without being burnt. Use capers only if you like them – they are an acquired taste.

1	Organic or free range chicken, weighing about 1.35 kg/3 lb	1
3 tbsp	Extra virgin olive oil	3 tbsp
2 tbsp	Lemon juice	2 tbsp
1	Garlic clove, crushed	1
2 tsp	Dijon mustard	2 tsp
	Sea salt and freshly ground black pepper	
110 g	Quinoa	4 oz
300 ml	Chicken stock (see page 159)	½ pint
1 tbsp	Finely grated lemon rind	1 tbsp
1 tbsp	Capers, rinsed (optional)	1 tbsp
3 tbsp	Sage leaves, finely sliced	3 tbsp
1 tbsp	Slivered almonds	1 tbsp
2	Whole lemons	2

Preheat the oven to 200°C/400°F/Gas Mark 6.

Joint the chicken into eight pieces. Cut off the wing tips and discard. Place the chicken joints in an ovenproof dish. Whisk together two tablespoons of olive oil, the lemon juice, crushed garlic, mustard and seasoning. Pour over the chicken, making sure it is all well coated. Bake in the preheated oven for ten minutes, then turn over and bake on the other side for another ten minutes.

Meanwhile, wash the quinoa, drain thoroughly, then put in a saucepan with the stock. Bring to the boil, lower the heat, cover and simmer for 20 minutes until tender and the liquid is absorbed. You may have to add a little more stock or water to prevent it drying out.

Heat the rest of the olive oil in a large frying pan over medium heat. Add the grated lemon rind, capers (if using), sage leaves and slivered almonds, and cook for 5 minutes or until the almonds are just beginning to turn colour. Add this mixture to the quinoa and mix together well. Keep warm while you finish off the chicken.

Preheat the grill. Transfer the chicken joints to the grill, draining off any fat that has accumulated. Cut the lemons in half and add them to the grill. Grill the chicken and lemons until crisp, turning once. Be careful not to let the chicken burn.

Serve the chicken pieces on a bed of lemon quinoa, and garnish with the grilled lemon halves.

Serves 4-5   **Time taken: 45 minutes**

Per serving
Calories 510kcals; Protein 38g; Carbohydrates 21g; Dietary Fibre 3g; Sugar – Total 1g; Fat – Total 30g; Saturated Fat 7g; Vitamin C 19mg; Magnesium 85mg

> Quinoa is not only delicious but a rich source of protein and minerals, especially magnesium and calcium. However, you could substitute barley or brown rice for the quinoa.

ROAST GUINEA FOWL WITH WALNUT SAUCE

Protein 36%   GI: low
Carbohydrate 11%   GL: low
Fat 53%

Guinea fowl makes a gamey, flavoursome change from chicken. This walnut sauce is based on those used in Iranian and other Middle Eastern cuisines, but without using hard-to-find ingredients.

1	Guinea fowl, about 1.6 kg/3½ lb	1
	Sea salt and freshly ground black pepper	
2 tbsp	Extra virgin olive oil	2 tbsp
60 g	Walnuts	2 oz
200 ml	Soya, rice or nut milk	7 fl oz
1 tsp	Cornflour	1 tsp
1	Small onion, peeled and finely chopped	1
3	Garlic cloves, peeled and finely chopped	3
150 ml	Dry white wine	¼ pint

	Freshly grated nutmeg	
1 tsp	Fresh thyme leaves	1 tsp
4 tbsp	Natural live yoghurt	4 tbsp

Preheat the oven to 200°C/400°F/Gas Mark 6.

Lightly season the guinea fowl with salt and pepper, place in a roasting tin on its side and pour over the olive oil (this is needed as guinea fowl can be quite dry). Roast for 20 minutes, then turn over and baste the other side and roast for another 20 minutes. Then turn the bird breast up and cook for another 20 minutes. Remove from the oven and leave to cool on a plate. Set aside the roasting pan and its juices.

Meanwhile, chop the walnuts roughly and put in a small bowl. Heat the milk and pour over the walnuts. Leave to infuse for half an hour, then strain and set the walnuts aside. Mix the milk with the cornflour and set that aside too.

When the guinea fowl has cooled sufficiently to handle, joint it into four pieces and place the pieces in a baking dish. Return to the oven for ten minutes while you prepare the sauce.

For the sauce, pour off the fat from the roasting tin, leaving a couple of spoonsful of juices. Set over a gentle heat and cook the chopped onion and garlic until tender but not browned. Add the white wine and continue cooking, scraping up any bits from the bottom of the pan. Finally add the milk and cornflour mixture, and cook, stirring, until the sauce has thickened. Add the nutmeg and thyme and adjust the seasoning if necessary. Cook for a further 5 minutes, then add the chopped soaked walnuts. Off the heat, stir in the yoghurt.

Serve the guinea fowl either with the sauce poured over, or handed round separately, accompanied by a selection of green vegetables.

Serves 4   **Time taken: 1½ hours**

Per serving
Calories 368kcals; Protein 31g; Carbohydrates 8g; Dietary Fibre 1g; Sugar – Total 3g; Fat – Total 21g; Saturated Fat 3g; Vitamin C 4mg; Magnesium 62mg

Any nuts could be used here in place of the walnuts. Try ground almonds or cashews.

TURKEY WITH FENNEL AND CASHEW CREAM

Protein 44%   GI: low
Carbohydrate 19%   GL: low
Fat 37%

This smooth creamy sauce gives the turkey an unusual aniseed flavour. Celery is a good substitute if you can't find fennel. This dish is a good balance of protein, carbohydrate and fat. Serve it with vegetables on the side, such as carrots and cabbage.

1 tbsp	Extra virgin olive oil	1 tbsp
350 g	Turkey meat, breast or thigh, cut into 2.5 cm/1 inch cubes	12 oz
1	Small onion, sliced	1
1-2	Fennel bulbs, sliced horizontally, reserving the fronds for garnish (about 8-10 oz/225-285 g)	1-2
1 tbsp	Plain or gluten-free white flour	1 tbsp
200 ml	Chicken stock	7 fl oz
1 tsp	Fresh thyme leaves, chopped	1 tsp
	Sea salt and freshly ground black pepper to taste	
60 g	Cashew nuts	2 oz
100 ml	Water	3½ fl oz

Preheat the oven to 170°C/325°F/Gas Mark 3.

Heat the oil in a frying pan over a medium heat, add the turkey and cook quite briskly until brown all over. Using a slotted spoon, transfer to an ovenproof casserole. Add the onion and fennel to the pan and cook for about 10 minutes, stirring occasionally.

Stir in the flour, then gradually add the stock, stirring all the time. Bring to a gentle boil, add the thyme, salt and pepper. Pour over the turkey. Cover and cook in the oven for 30 minutes. Meanwhile chop the fennel fronds for use as a garnish. Blend the cashew nuts and water together until smooth to make a thick cream.

Take the casserole out of the oven, stir in the cashew cream, cover and continue cooking for about 15-20 minutes, or until the turkey is tender. Serve sprinkled with the chopped fennel fronds.

Serves 4   **Time taken: 1¼ hours**

Per serving
Calories 254kcals; Protein 28g; Carbohydrates 12g; Dietary

Fibre 3g; Sugar – Total 2g; Fat – Total 11g; Saturated Fat 2g; Vitamin C 9mg; Magnesium 59mg

Fennel contains the antioxidant flavonoid quercetin. It can also be useful for indigestion and spasms of the digestive tract. It also helps expel phlegm from the lungs.

CINNAMON SMOKED DUCK

Protein 46%
Carbohydrate 3%
Fat 51%

GI: very low
GL: very low

This is the Chinese method for home smoking, and is surprisingly straightforward, though it can create a lot of smoke in your kitchen, so turn on the exhaust fan before you start. Smoked food is thought to be carcinogenic, but the duck is smoked for quite a short time just to impart flavour, and because you use only the duck breasts, the smoking takes much less time than if you were smoking a whole duck. Although there is white rice and sugar in the recipe, you don't eat them, so it's a good way to get rid of these nutrient-poor foods that you may have in your store cupboard.

4	Duck breasts	4
1 tsp	Coarse sea salt	1 tsp
1 tsp	Szechuan peppercorns	1 tsp
90 g	Uncooked white rice	3 oz
90 g	Sugar	3 oz
2	Cinnamon sticks, broken up into small pieces	2
3	Star anise	3
2 tbsp	Chinese black tea leaves, such as Lapsang Souchong	2 tbsp
6	Bok choy, halved	6
2 tbsp	Tamari	2 tbsp
2 tsp	Oriental sesame oil	2 tsp

Wipe the duck breasts and prick them two or three times with a sharp fork. Crush the salt and Szechuan pepper and toast them in a wok. Cool, then rub all over the duck breasts.

Fill the wok about one third full with water and place a rack over it. Put the duck breasts on the rack, cover and steam for 20-30 minutes, depending on the thickness of the breasts.

To prepare the wok for smoking, wash it out, dry and line with a double thickness of foil. Mix together the rice, sugar, cinnamon, star anise and tea leaves and spread in the bottom of the wok. Place the rack on top and arrange the duck breasts on it. Put the lid on and seal the edge with a strip of foil. Turn the heat to medium-high and place the wok on the heat. Once it has begun to smoke, which you will smell rather than see, resist the temptation to have a look, and leave the wok on the heat for 10-15 minutes. Remove from the heat and leave to stand for another 15 minutes.

While the duck is standing, steam the bok choy over boiling water for 5 minutes. Place on individual plates. Remove the duck from the wok, slice each breast diagonally into three or four slices and arrange on the bed of bok choy. Sprinkle with tamari and oriental sesame oil.

The smoked duck breasts can also be served cold or at room temperature, thinly sliced.

Serves 4   **Time taken: 1 hour 20 minutes**

Per serving
Calories 279kcals; Protein 32g; Carbohydrates 2g; Dietary Fibre 1g; Sugar – Total 0g; Fat – Total 15g; Saturated Fat 4g; Vitamin C 25mg; Magnesium 13mg

Duck is known to be a fatty meat, but the initial pricking of the skin and steaming renders quite a lot of the fat, and if you are concerned you can always discard the skin before eating. Interestingly, nearly half the fat in duck skin is of the mono-unsaturated variety, so it may be less harmful than is generally supposed. Duck meat supplies some 'haem' iron which is easily absorbed, useful for those who do not eat red meat, the other good supplier of haem iron.

FISH

As a nutritional therapist, I find myself constantly advising people to eat more fish, and specifically oily fish. The dilemma is: which fish is it safe and/or environmentally friendly to eat? My answer is that as far as white fish are concerned, our cod stocks are now seriously depleted, and it is better to substitute hake or haddock, both of which appear to be in better supply. As for oily fish, the large carnivorous fish such as tuna and swordfish at the top of the food chain tend to have accumulated more mercury than smaller fry such as mackerel and sardines, so I would opt for the latter. As for salmon, farmed salmon is now very polluted, due to overcrowding and poor farming practices. Yet I still feel that if you cannot afford organic or wild salmon, both of which are very expensive, eating farmed salmon once a week or so is better than eating no oily fish at all. Canned salmon is an option, as it is usually wild oceanic salmon. Another solution may be to choose rainbow trout, which, although it contains less omega-3's in it than salmon, is generally farmed in cleaner conditions than salmon.

COCONUT FISH CURRY

Protein 57%
Carbohydrate 12%
Fat 31%

GI: low
GL: low

Monkfish works best in this curry, as it has a good, firm texture and does not fall apart as easily as other white fish.

2 tsp	Cumin seeds	2 tsp
2 tsp	Coriander seeds	2 tsp
1/2 tsp	Fenugreek seeds	1/2 tsp
1 tbsp	Coconut oil	1 tbsp
1	Cinnamon stick	1
1	Star anise	1
2	Organic limes, finely grated zest and juice	2
1	Can coconut milk (400 ml)	1
675 g	Firm white fish, such as monkfish, hake or haddock, cut into 2.5 cm/1 inch cubes	1½ lb
	Fresh coriander leaves, for garnish	

In an electric grinder, grind the cumin seeds, coriander seeds and fenugreek seeds to a powder. Heat the coconut oil in a large frying pan over medium heat. Add the ground spices, cinnamon stick, star anise and the grated lime zest. Cook, stirring, for a couple of minutes until the spices start to release their fragrance. Pour in the coconut milk, bring to the boil, then reduce the heat and simmer for 5 minutes to allow the flavours to meld.

Add the fish to the coconut sauce and simmer for about 8 minutes or until cooked through. Remove the cinnamon stick and star anise, and stir in the lime juice. You may not need all of it, so taste as you go – the lime and coconut should balance each other.

Serve garnished with coriander leaves and accompanied by brown rice or barley.

Serves 4   **Time taken: 25 minutes**

Per serving
Calories 227kcals; Protein 32g; Carbohydrates 7g; Dietary Fibre 2g; Sugar – Total 1g; Fat – Total 8g; Saturated Fat 4g; Vitamin C 15mg; Magnesium 99mg

This recipe contains coconut oil, cinnamon and fenugreek, all ingredients known to be beneficial for people with diabetes.

SALMON WITH MINTED PEA PURÉE AND ASPARAGUS

Protein 46%   GI: medium
Carbohydrate 17%   GL: low
Fat 37%

This is a dish with which to celebrate the arrival of summer. Unfortunately, though, the English asparagus season does not coincide with the pea harvest, so you will have to use either frozen peas or imported asparagus. I think I would opt for the former.

1	Leek, well washed and thinly sliced	1
15 g	Organic unsalted butter	½ oz
200 ml	Vegetable stock (see page 158)	7 fl oz
4	Fillets of wild or organic salmon, about 170 g/6 oz	4
350 g	Peas, frozen or freshly shelled (about 900 g/2 lb unshelled)	12 oz
6	Mint leaves, chopped	6
	Sea salt and freshly ground black pepper	
12	Asparagus tips	12

Place the leek, butter and stock in a saucepan over medium heat. Bring to a simmer, cover with a lid and cook over very low heat for 20 minutes, stirring once or twice.

Meanwhile, place each salmon fillet in a piece of foil, top each with a slice of lemon and a sprig of parsley, and wrap loosely, making sure that all the edges are sealed. Place under a hot grill for 15-20 minutes, depending on thickness, turning once.

While the salmon is cooking, add the peas and chopped mint to the leek mixture, cover and cook for 5 minutes. Remove the lid, and continue to cook until the peas are tender, about another 5 minutes. Drain, reserving the cooking liquid. Leave to cool a little, then tip into a blender or food processor together with about 3 tablespoons of the reserved liquid. Process until smooth, then season to taste and return to the pan to reheat gently.

Steam the asparagus tips over boiling water until done – 6 minutes if they are small.

To serve, place the pea purée on individual plates, unwrap the salmon and place on the purée. Garnish with the asparagus tips.

Serves 4   **Time taken: 45 minutes**

GRILLED TROUT WITH SALSA VERDE

Protein 31%   GI: low
Carbohydrate 4%   GL: low
Fat 65%

*Salsa verde is a wonderful Italian sauce, just right with grilled
trout, but it could equally well be served with grilled mackerel or
other strongly flavoured fish. It is traditionally made with a pestle
and mortar, but I'm afraid I cheat and use the food processor.*

1	Large bunch flat leaf parsley	1
8	Anchovy fillets, drained and chopped	8
2 tbsp	Capers, rinsed and drained	2 tbsp
2 tsp	Dry mustard powder	2 tsp
3	Garlic cloves, peeled and chopped	3
1	Lemon, juice only	1
2 tbsp	Fresh basil, chopped	2 tbsp
	Freshly ground black pepper	
8 tbsp	Extra virgin olive oil	8 tbsp
4	Whole trout, gutted, washed and with the fins cut off	4
1	Lemon, sliced	1

Remove the stems from the parsley, reserving a few for stuffing the
trout. Wash and chop the parsley leaves.

Place the anchovies, capers, mustard, garlic, lemon juice, parsley,
basil and pepper in the food processor, and process to a paste.
With the machine running, gradually pour in the olive oil, as for
mayonnaise. Taste and adjust seasoning. The salsa will separate on
standing, so leave in the food processor while you grill the trout,
then give it a final whizz just before serving to recombine.

Preheat the grill to high. Slash the trout 2-3 times on each side,
and tuck lemon slices and parsley stalks in the belly cavity.
Grill the trout for about 5 minutes per side, until crisp and sizzling.
Serve with the salsa verde.

Serves 4   **Time taken: 30 minutes**

Per serving
**Calories 553kcals; Protein 42g; Carbohydrates 6g; Dietary Fibre
2g; Sugar – Total 1g; Fat – Total 40g; Saturated Fat 7g; Vitamin
C 50mg; Magnesium 74mg**

Trout have less fat than other oily fish, so therefore less of the beneficial omega-3 fatty acids. However, they do contain some, and are also a very good source of potassium.

ROASTED MACKEREL WITH HORSERADISH CREAM

Protein 33%   GI: low
Carbohydrate 7%   GL: low
Fat 60%

Mackerel's pink, firm flesh is tasty, nutritious and inexpensive. The skin should shine – if it doesn't, don't buy it. It has a strong flavour which works well with robust accompaniments such as horseradish, and is one of the best sources of omega-3 fatty acids.

4	Whole fresh mackerel, gutted and with heads and fins removed	4
1	Organic lemon, grated zest and juice	1
2	Garlic cloves, peeled and finely chopped	2
	Cherry tomatoes on the vine	
1 tbsp	Extra virgin olive oil	1 tbsp
	Horseradish Cream:	
2-3 tbsp	Grated fresh horseradish	2-3 tbsp
2 tsp	Wine vinegar	2 tsp
1 tsp	Lemon juice	1 tsp
3 tsp	Prepared English mustard	3 tsp
1 tsp	Sea salt	1 tsp
	Freshly ground black pepper	
1 tsp	Concentrated apple juice	1 tsp
150 g	Natural live yoghurt	5 oz

Preheat the oven to 220°C/450°F/Gas Mark 7.

First make the Horseradish Cream: scrub the horseradish root well, peel and grate. Put the grated horseradish into a bowl with the vinegar, lemon juice, mustard, salt, freshly ground pepper and sugar. Fold in the yoghurt but do not overmix or the sauce will curdle. There will be more than enough for this recipe, but save the rest for another dish. It keeps for 2-3 days in the fridge.

Slash the mackerel 3 times on each side and rub the flesh with the lemon zest and garlic. Place on a baking tray and drizzle with the lemon juice. Arrange the tomatoes on the baking tray and drizzle with the olive oil. Bake in the preheated oven for 10 minutes, until the fish is cooked through and the skin is brown and crisp.

Serve the mackerel and tomatoes with the horseradish cream on the side. Steamed green beans make a good accompaniment.

Serves 4   **Time taken: 25 minutes**

Per serving
Calories 459kcals; Protein 38g; Carbohydrates 7g; Dietary Fibre 1g; Sugar – Total 2g; Fat – Total 30g; Saturated Fat 7g; Vitamin C 18mg; Magnesium 147mg

To prepare fresh horseradish, scrub the root well, remove the skin with a vegetable peeler, then grate the white flesh. Avoid touching your eyes whilst preparing horseradish, as it is very pungent and can sting them. This property is what makes it so good for clearing stuffy noses and blocked sinuses. If you can't get fresh horseradish, substitute prepared horseradish and reduce the amount of yoghurt.

VEGETABLES AND SALADS

Vegetables should be the mainstay of any diet, accounting for at least half of every meal, but too often they are treated as an afterthought. Eating them raw in salads, or as juices, is the way to get maximum benefit from all the nutrition they provide. The next best thing is to steam them, as few of their nutrients are lost this way – even the water over which they have been steamed can be used as a vegetable stock, or even drunk as a light soup.

Microwaving vegetables, on the other hand, can cause them to lose 97% of the antioxidants that help us fight cancer and heart disease, according to the *Journal of the Science of Food and Agriculture*. Deep-frying is just as harmful, as it produces free radicals which destroy essential fats in food and can damage cells. Ironically it is the polyunsaturated oils that oxidise most rapidly, becoming dangerous 'trans' fats. So it is safer to use butter or coconut oil, which are saturated fats, or olive oil which is monounsaturated. When stir frying, keep the frying part to a minimum, adding liquid as soon in the process as possible to cut down the frying time.

Here is a handful of tasty vegetable dishes, intended to be accompaniments to protein foods such as fish, chicken or beans, although some of them would work as light meals in their own right.

BRAISED KALE

Protein 11%
Carbohydrate 26%
Fat 63%

GI: low
GL: low

This is a quick and tasty way to cook kale, which some people find a dull vegetable. It's anything but dull like this, though. Alternative ways to cook kale are to boil it just in the water clinging to the leaves, for 6 minutes, or stir-fry it with ginger, garlic and sesame seeds.

450 g	Kale	1 lb
2 tbsp	Extra virgin olive oil	2 tbsp
2	Garlic cloves, chopped	2
100 ml	Vegetable stock (see page 158)	3½ fl oz
2 tbsp	Shoyu sauce	2 tbsp
2 tbsp	Rice vinegar	2 tbsp
1	Lemon, juice and finely grated rind	1
	Sea salt and freshly ground black pepper to taste	
1 tbsp	Flaked almonds, lightly toasted	1 tbsp

Wash the kale, separate the stems from the leaves and chop both coarsely, discarding the very woody parts of the stems. Heat the oil in a wok or large sauté pan over medium heat. Sauté the garlic and kale stems for 3 minutes, then add the kale leaves, vegetable stock and shoyu. Cover and cook until the kale is tender, about 5-7 minutes. Remove from the heat and add the vinegar, lemon juice and rind, and seasoning to taste. Toss well. Serve topped with toasted flaked almonds.

Serves 4   Time taken: 20 minutes

Per serving
Calories 150kcals; Protein 4g; Carbohydrates 11g; Dietary Fibre 3g; Sugar – Total 3g; Fat – Total 11g; Saturated Fat 1g; Vitamin C 53mg; Magnesium 28mg

Kale is rich in potassium and folate, calcium, thiamine and vitamin B6. In addition, it is positively bristling with cancer-fighting phytochemicals and glucosinolates. Kale consumption has been linked with lower incidences of colon and bladder cancer.

BROCCOLI WITH GARLIC

Protein 18%
Carbohydrate 30%
Fat 52%

GI: low
GL: low

This is an oriental way of cooking broccoli which can also be used with cauliflower. The broccoli is steamed for a few minutes first which ensures it is tender before the final stir-frying. Don't throw away the broccoli stems – either peel, cut into discs and steam together with the florets, or use raw in salads.

1 kg	Broccoli	2 lb 2 oz
2 tbsp	Extra virgin olive oil	2 tbsp
1 tsp	Fresh ginger root, peeled and finely chopped	1 tsp
2	Garlic cloves, peeled and finely chopped	2
1/2	Fresh red chilli, deseeded and finely chopped (optional)	1/2
	Freshly ground black pepper	
2 tbsp	Pine nuts	2 tbsp
2 tsp	Tamari	2 tsp

Wash the broccoli and divide into florets. Steam over boiling water for 2 minutes only, then set aside.

Heat the olive oil in a wok over medium heat. Add the ginger, garlic and chilli (if using), stir once, then add the broccoli florets. Stir fry for about 4 minutes, and season with pepper. Toss in the pine nuts and serve sprinkled with tamari.

Variations: Try this with sesame seeds instead of pine nuts.
Serves 4   **Time taken: 10 minutes**

Per serving
Calories 143kcals; Protein 7g; Carbohydrates 12g; Dietary Fibre 6g; Sugar – Total 4g; Fat – Total 9g; Saturated Fat 1g; Vitamin C 172mg; Magnesium 62mg

> Broccoli is an amazingly nutritious vegetable. It contains twice as much vitamin C as an orange; it has almost as much calcium as whole milk – and the calcium is better absorbed; and it contains selenium, a mineral that has been found to have anti-cancer and anti-viral properties. It is also a modest source of vitamin A and alpha-tocopherol vitamin E.

GREEN VEGETABLE STIR FRY

Protein 12%　　　　　　　　　　　　　　　　GI: very low
Carbohydrate 48%　　　　　　　　　　　　　GL: low
Fat 40%

This recipe is an adaptation of one by Dr Mercola, a doctor with quite radical views who runs one of the best independent health sites on the internet, www.mercola.com.

2 tbsp	Coconut oil	2 tbsp
2	Garlic cloves, peeled and crushed	2
2	Medium leeks, washed and sliced	2
450 g	Brussels sprouts, washed and quartered	1 lb
1 tsp	Fresh chopped rosemary	1 tsp
450 g	Bunch of kale, stems removed and coarsely chopped	1 lb
4 tbsp	Water	4 tbsp
2 tbsp	Dijon mustard	2 tbsp
	Freshly ground black pepper	

Heat a wok or heavy saucepan with a cover over high heat. Add oil and garlic and stir for a few seconds. Then add the sliced leeks. Stir-fry, stirring constantly, for about 2-3 minutes or until the leeks start to wilt. Add the Brussels sprouts and rosemary and stir-fry for 2-3 minutes. Reduce the heat to medium, add the chopped kale and water, stirring to combine. Cover and steam for 3-5 minutes, until the vegetables are tender. Remove the cover and stir in the Dijon mustard. Season with freshly ground black pepper. Remove to a serving dish and serve immediately.

Serves 4　　　　　　　　　　　　　　**Time taken: 15 minutes**

Per serving
Calories 171kcals; Protein 6g; Carbohydrates 23g; Dietary Fibre 6g; Sugar – Total 8g; Fat – Total 9g; Saturated Fat 6g; Vitamin C 119mg; Magnesium 54mg

Kale contains lutein and zeaxanthin, phytonutrients which protect the eyes from macular degeneration. Leeks, being a member of the onion family, contain quercetin which protects against heart disease. So this mixture of vegetables is particularly good for people with diabetes whose heart and eye health are especially at risk.

SPICED RED CABBAGE WITH PRUNES

Protein 6%
Carbohydrate 56%
Fat 38%

GI: low
GL: low

This recipe is brilliant because it contains not only cinnamon, the virtues of which I have mentioned elsewhere, but also juniper berries. Juniper berries have the reputation of being able to regulate blood sugar. I have not found any clinical trials to support this theory, but it's always worth paying attention to folk medicine.

675 g	Red cabbage	1½ lb
225 g	Onions	8 oz
45 g	Butter	1½ oz
½ tsp	Ground cinnamon	½ tsp
4	Whole cloves	4
½ tsp	Freshly grated nutmeg	½ tsp
½ tsp	Crushed juniper berries	½ tsp
110 g	Dried, ready-to-eat prunes	4 oz
3 tbsp	Concentrated apple juice	3 tbsp
3 tbsp	Red wine vinegar	3 tbsp
	Sea salt and freshly ground black pepper to taste	

Preheat the oven to 150°C/300°F/Gas Mark 2.

Shred the cabbage finely, discarding the core. Place half the cabbage in the bottom of a casserole. Place half the onions on top and then all the spices and the prunes.

Add half the butter in knobs and season with salt and pepper. Top with the rest of the cabbage and the onions. Mix the vinegar and apple juice concentrate together and pour over the cabbage. Top with the rest of the butter.

Cover with a lid and bake for 3 hours, stirring occasionally, until tender. Taste and adjust the seasoning. Serve hot.

Serves 4   **Time taken: 3¼ hours**

Per serving
Calories 217kcals; Protein 3g; Carbohydrates 32g; Dietary Fibre 6g; Sugar – Total 22g; Fat – Total 10g; Saturated Fat 6g; Vitamin C 62mg; Magnesium 31mg

Red cabbage has all the virtues of green cabbage, with the added advantage of lycopene, which is responsible for the red colouring, also found in tomatoes. Research has found that higher intakes of this antioxidant in the diet are associated with lower levels of heart disease, especially in men.

STIR-FRIED BEAN SPROUTS

Protein 18% GI: very low
Carbohydrate 42% GL: very low
Fat 40%

Mung bean sprouts are specified here, but feel free to use any sprouted beans or seeds in this stir-fry.

450 g	Mung bean sprouts	1 lb
1 tbsp	Extra virgin olive oil	1 tbsp
3	Spring onions, split lengthways and cut into 2.5 cm/1 inch lengths	3
1 tbsp	Fresh ginger root, peeled and finely chopped	1 tbsp
½ tsp	Freshly ground black pepper	½ tsp
	Tamari	

Wash, drain and dry the bean sprouts on kitchen paper.

Heat the olive oil in a wok over medium-high heat. Add the spring onions and ginger, and stir-fry for a few seconds. Then add the bean sprouts and stir-fry for 1 minute. Do not overcook – sprouts should remain crunchy but lose their raw bean taste.

Season to taste with pepper, and sprinkle with tamari. Mix well and serve.

Serves 4 **Time taken: 10 minutes**

Per serving
Calories 75kcals; Protein 4g; Carbohydrates 9g; Dietary Fibre 2g; Sugar – Total 4g; Fat – Total 4g; Saturated Fat 1g; Vitamin C 17mg; Magnesium 27mg

Mung beans are small dried green beans with yellow flesh. Like all beans, they are rich in protein, calcium, phosphorus and iron, but they are mainly grown for sprouting. Mung bean sprouts have long been a familiar ingredient in many Asian dishes. Traditional Chinese medicine maintains that mung beans have a "heat-clearing, toxin-resolving" effect that eases conditions such as diarrhoea. They should be of particular interest to people with diabetes because they contain chiro-inositol, an ingredient also present in buckwheat, which may prompt cells to become more insulin-sensitive.

WARM EAST-WEST SALAD

Protein 14%
Carbohydrate 50%
Fat 36%

GI: medium
GL: low

The style of this warm salad is oriental, but the vegetables come straight from an English garden.

225 g	Carrots	8 oz
225 g	French beans	8 oz
1	Cauliflower weighing about 450 g/1 lb	1
1/2	Fresh red chilli, deseeded and finely chopped	1/2
1 tsp	Apple juice concentrate	1 tsp
2 tbsp	Shoyu sauce	2 tbsp
1 tbsp	Oriental sesame oil	1 tbsp
1 tbsp	Sesame seeds, toasted	1 tbsp
	For the broth:	
600 ml	Vegetable stock (see page 158)	1 pint
1	Medium onion, peeled and finely chopped	1
1 tsp	Ginger root, grated	1 tsp
3	Sprigs of thyme	3
1	Lime, juice only	1

Put all the ingredients for the broth into a pan, bring to the boil, cover and simmer for 5 minutes. Leave to infuse while you prepare the vegetables.

Cut the carrots into sticks about 5 cm/2 inches long, and cut the beans the same length. Separate the cauliflower into small florets. Strain the broth and return it to the pan. Bring to the boil and cook the vegetables in it for 3-4 minutes – not more, as they should retain some 'bite'. When cooked, drain the vegetables, reserving 3 tablespoons of the cooking broth. Place the vegetables in a serving bowl. Reserve 3 tablespoons of the cooking broth.

For the dressing, whisk together the reserved cooking broth, chopped chilli, apple juice concentrate, shoyu sauce and sesame oil.

Pour this over the vegetables and sprinkle with sesame seeds.
Serve warm or at room temperature.

Serves 4   **Time taken: 20 minutes**

Per serving
Calories 123kcals; Protein 5g; Carbohydrates 17g; Dietary Fibre
7g; Sugar – Total 6g; Fat – Total 5g; Saturated Fat 1g; Vitamin C
69mg; Magnesium 34mg

VEGETABLES IN CURRIED COCONUT CREAM

Protein 10%   GI: medium
Carbohydrate 34%   GL: very low
Fat 56%

*I serve this delicious vegetable mixture with plain brown rice, but
you could serve it as an accompaniment to a Thai meal. Root
vegetables increase their glycaemic index as they cook, so serve this
when the carrots and celeriac still have some 'bite'.*

1 tbsp	Coconut oil	1 tbsp
1	Large onion, thinly sliced	1
2	Garlic cloves, crushed	2
2.5 cm	Piece of ginger root, peeled and finely chopped	1 inch
1 tbsp	Curry paste	1 tbsp
1 tsp	Ground turmeric	1 tsp
¹/₂ tsp	Chopped fresh chilli	¹/₂ tsp
	Sea salt and freshly ground black pepper to taste	
300 ml	Vegetable stock (see page 158)	¹/₂ pint
550 g	Celeriac, peeled and cut into 2.5 cm/1 inch cubes	1¹/₄ lb
2	Carrots, sliced	2
110 g	French beans, cut into 5 cm/2 inch lengths	4 oz
200 ml	Coconut cream	7 fl oz
	Fresh coriander, chopped, for garnish	

Heat the coconut oil in a large saucepan over low heat and add the
onion, garlic and ginger. Cook for about 5 minutes, until softened
but not brown. Stir in the curry paste, turmeric, chilli and

seasoning. Add the stock, bring to the boil, and add the celeriac, carrots and green beans. Cover and cook over gentle heat for 10 minutes. Stir in the coconut cream and continue cooking for another few minutes, until heated through and the vegetables are just tender but still resistant to the bite. Serve garnished with chopped fresh coriander.

Serves 4   **Time taken: 20 minutes**

Per serving
Calories 151kcals; Protein 4g; Carbohydrates 13g; Dietary Fibre 4g; Sugar – Total 5g; Fat – Total 10g; Saturated Fat 3g; Vitamin C 18mg; Magnesium 36mg

AVOCADO, GRAPEFRUIT AND ALFALFA SALAD

Protein 5%   GI: very low
Carbohydrate 21%   GL: very low
Fat 74%

This started out as an attempt to design a salad full of foods rich in vitamin E. However, it turned out to be too high in fat, as vitamin E is a fat-soluble vitamin. So I added grapefruit to cut the richness. It still has quite a lot of fat, although mostly monounsaturated, so I would serve it with plain grilled fish or chicken and a steamed green vegetable.

2	Avocados	2
1/2	Lemon, juice only	1/2
2	Pink grapefruit	2
	Alfalfa sprouts, a handful	
30 g	Sunflower seeds, toasted	1 oz
	Vinaigrette made with walnut or avocado oil (see page 162)	

Peel and slice the avocados. Brush the cut surfaces with lemon juice to prevent discoloration. Peel the grapefruit, removing all the pith, and slice thinly into segments.

Fan out the avocado slices and grapefruit segments on individual plates, and put a mound of alfalfa sprouts on each serving. Garnish with toasted sunflower seeds and dress with walnut or avocado oil vinaigrette.

Serves 4   **Time taken: 15 minutes**

Per serving
Calories 372kcals; Protein 5g; Carbohydrates 21g; Dietary Fibre
8g; Sugar – Total 9g; Fat – Total 33g; Saturated Fat 4g; Vitamin
C 60mg; Magnesium 70mg

Avocados are nutritionally rich and should not be avoided on
account of their fat content. They contain 4 times as much
monounsaturated, and 4.5 times as much polyunsaturated fat
(the good kinds) as saturated fat (the 'bad' kind). They are also
a good source of minerals, particularly potassium, and most of
the B vitamins which we need for energy. As for grapefruit,
recent research has shown that grapefruit really does contribute
to weight loss, by moderating both insulin and blood glucose.
It appears that grapefruit contains enzymes that help control
insulin spikes after a meal. This frees the digestive system to
process food more efficiently, which means that fewer nutrients
are stored as fat.

BEAN AND SEED SPROUTS WITH AVOCADO DRESSING

Protein 12%   GI: very low
Carbohydrate 41%   GL: very low
Fat 47%

*Use whatever sprouts you have available for this salad – below are
only suggestions. Bioforce do little packets of mixed seeds for
sprouting – these are ideal (see Useful Addresses). If you don't have
a juicer with which to make the carrot juice, cook and purée a
couple of carrots and thin the purée with a little water.*

30 g	Mung bean sprouts	1 oz
30 g	Sprouted chickpeas	1 oz
30 g	Alfalfa sprouts	1 oz
15 g	Sprouted fenugreek seeds	1/2 oz
1	Red pepper, deseeded and thinly sliced	1
2	Tomatoes, peeled, deseeded and diced	2
1/2	Cucumber, peeled and sliced	1/2

1	Ripe avocado	1
1 tbsp	Lime juice	1 tbsp
4 tbsp	Carrot juice, preferably freshly made	4 tbsp
1	Garlic clove, finely chopped	1
	Sea salt and freshly ground black pepper	

For the dressing, peel and roughly chop the avocado. Put all the ingredients in the blender and blend to mix. The avocado should not discolour due to the lime juice.

For the salad, mix all the ingredients. Toss with the avocado dressing and serve.

Serves 4   **Time taken: 15 minutes**

Per serving
Calories 147kcals; Protein 5g; Carbohydrates 17g; Dietary Fibre 6g; Sugar – Total 4g; Fat – Total 8g; Saturated Fat 1g; Vitamin C 75mg; Magnesium 41mg

Mung beans are thought to be beneficial as an antidiabetic, low glycaemic index food, rich in antioxidants. I have included sprouted fenugreek seeds as they have similar properties.

CHINESE-STYLE BROCCOLI SALAD

Protein 11%
Carbohydrate 29%
Fat 60%

GI: very low
GL: very low

The origins of this recipe lie in Elaine Bruce's Living Foods for Radiant Health. *Elaine runs the Living Foods Clinic in Ludlow, the theory behind which is that only by eating raw foods can we obtain all the nutrients we need for maximum health. This dictum is quite hard for most people to follow, but it is certainly wise to incorporate a generous proportion of raw vegetables into our diet. Elaine's broccoli salad incorporates raw peppers and no dressing. This is my not quite authentic version.*

1	Red pepper	1
1	Yellow pepper	1
450 g	Raw broccoli florets, finely chopped	1 lb
4	Courgettes, grated	4

	Dressing:	
1 tbsp	Toasted sesame oil	1 tbsp
2 tbsp	Extra virgin olive oil	2 tbsp
2 tbsp	Fresh lemon juice	2 tbsp
2	Garlic cloves, peeled and crushed	2
1 tbsp	Fresh root ginger, peeled and grated	1 tbsp
	Sea salt and freshly ground black pepper	
	To serve: Green salad leaves	

Grill the peppers under a hot grill, turning from time to time, until just charred. Leave to cool, then skin, deseed and cut into strips.

Save a few tiny leaves and florets of broccoli for decoration. Mix the chopped broccoli with the grated courgettes. Whisk together all the ingredients for the dressing, then stir into the broccoli and courgette, mixing thoroughly to balance the flavours. Turn the salad onto a dish of green leaves and decorate with strips of red and yellow pepper.

Serves 4   **Time taken: 35 minutes**

Per serving
Calories 154kcals; Protein 5g; Carbohydrates 12g; Dietary Fibre 5g; Sugar – Total 4g; Fat – Total 11g; Saturated Fat 2g; Vitamin C 230mg; Magnesium 46mg

This salad is a rich source of beta-carotene, vitamin B6, folic acid and particularly vitamin C, of which it has a staggering 230 mg, which is nearly ten times the daily estimated average requirement (EAR) for this vitamin.

FENNEL AND RED CABBAGE SALAD
WITH PUMPKIN SEEDS

Protein 15%   GI: very low
Carbohydrate 40%   GL: very low
Fat 45%

Raw fennel is my absolutely favourite vegetable. If you can get hold of organic fennel, you will notice that its aniseed taste is much more pronounced than that of the conventionally grown vegetable.

2	Fennel bulbs	2
1/2	Small red cabbage (about 225 g/8 oz)	1/2
3	Spring onions, finely chopped	3
2 tbsp	Pumpkin seeds	2 tbsp
2 tbsp	Natural live yoghurt	2 tbsp
1 tbsp	Extra virgin olive oil	1 tbsp
	Squeeze of lemon juice	
	Sea salt and freshly ground black pepper	

Trim the fennel, reserving the frondy tops. Cut vertically into quarters, then slice as finely as possible. Shred the cabbage as finely as possible. Put the vegetables into a salad bowl and add the chopped spring onions.

Toast the pumpkin seeds in a small dry pan until they begin to give off their aroma, but be careful not to let them get too dark.

For the dressing, mix together the yoghurt and olive oil, sharpen with a little lemon juice and season to taste. Stir the dressing into the fennel mixture until well combined.

Chop the fennel fronds and use them to garnish the salad, together with the toasted pumpkin seeds.

Serves 4   **Time taken: 20 minutes**

Per serving
Calories 129kcals; Protein 5g; Carbohydrates 14g; Dietary Fibre 5g; Sugar – Total 3g; Fat – Total 7g; Saturated Fat 1g; Vitamin C 48mg; Magnesium 68mg

Besides its other virtues, fennel contains a good range of microminerals – those minerals of which we only need a small amount, such as selenium, iron, manganese and molybdenum. Molybdenum is needed by some of the enzyme systems in the body that are involved in detoxification.

GREEK MUSHROOM SALAD

Protein 7%   GI: very low
Carbohydrate 18%   GL: very low
Fat 75%

Otherwise known as 'champignons à la grècque', this is a French rather than a Greek salad.

350 g	Small button mushrooms	12 oz
100 ml	Dry white wine	3¹/₂ fl oz
100 ml	Water	3¹/₂ fl oz
100 ml	Extra virgin olive oil	3¹/₂ fl oz
1	Lemon, juice only	1
1	Bay leaf	1
2 tbsp	Chopped onion	2 tbsp
2 tsp	Fresh thyme leaves	2 tsp
	Pinch of ground coriander	
1 tsp	Fennel seeds	1 tsp
	Sea salt and freshly ground black pepper	

Wipe the mushrooms, but do not peel them. If the mushrooms are very small, leave them whole. Otherwise, cut them in half or into quarters, depending on their size. Put all the remaining ingredients into a saucepan, bring to the boil and simmer them for 5 minutes. Add the mushrooms and simmer for another 5 minutes. Let the mushrooms cool in the liquid before placing in a bowl to serve.

Serves 4   **Time taken: 20 minutes**

Per serving
Calories 142kcals; Protein 3g; Carbohydrates 5g; Dietary Fibre 2g; Sugar – Total 2g; Fat – Total 12g; Saturated Fat 2g; Vitamin C 8mg; Magnesium 14mg

Because mushrooms contain chromium, it is important for people with diabetes to include them in their diet, as it is one of the major components of glucose tolerance factor, a molecule that improves insulin's ability to lower blood sugar levels. Chromium also helps to reduce sugar cravings.

LIME-SCENTED CARROT AND CUMIN SALAD

Protein 4%
Carbohydrate 39%
Fat 57%

GI: very low
GL: very low

This is a good way to use the larger, older carrots. Given this treatment they appear to regain their youth.

2 tsp	Cumin seeds	2 tsp
3 tbsp	Extra virgin olive oil	3 tbsp
1	Organic lime, grated zest and juice	1
	Sea salt and freshly ground black pepper	
3-4	Large maincrop carrots, peeled and finely grated (about 675 g/1½ lb)	3-4
1	Red onion, peeled and thinly sliced into rings	1
1 tbsp	Coriander leaves, chopped	1 tbsp

First, dry fry the cumin seeds in a small pan until they begin to release their aroma. Be careful as they can jump out of the pan when they get hot. Set aside.

Whisk together the olive oil, lime juice and zest, and seasoning. Put the carrots and onions into a salad bowl, toss with the dressing, then stir in the toasted cumin seeds. Garnish with chopped coriander.

Serves 4   **Time taken: 20 minutes**

Per serving
Calories 165kcals; Protein 2g; Carbohydrates 17g; Dietary Fibre 5g; Sugar – Total 10g; Fat – Total 11g; Saturated Fat 2g; Vitamin C 20mg; Magnesium 24mg

Raw carrots have a GI of 16 or thereabouts, but as much as 49 after cooking. Since they are our richest source of the antioxidant beta-carotene and other carotenoids, which help to provide protection against free radical damage, it is a good idea for people with diabetes to eat them regularly.

PINK AND PURPLE SALAD

Protein 5%   GI: very low
Carbohydrate 31%   GL: very low
Fat 64%

I designed this salad to take advantage of the beautiful purple curly kale when it comes into season in the winter. If you can't find it, use ordinary green kale, which has the same nutritive properties.

2	Small raw beetroot	2
1	Pink or red grapefruit	1
100 g	Purple curly kale, washed and torn into bite-sized pieces, woody stems discarded	3½ oz
12	Radishes, preferably French breakfast variety, sliced	12
	For the dressing:	
4 tbsp	Orange juice	4 tbsp
1 tsp	Finely grated orange zest from an organic orange	1 tsp
4 tbsp	Extra virgin olive oil	4 tbsp
1 tbsp	Finely grated fresh ginger root	1 tbsp
2 tbsp	Chopped parsley	2 tbsp
	Sea salt and freshly ground black pepper	

Peel and grate the beetroot. Whisk together all the dressing ingredients and stir half the dressing into the beetroot. Leave for an hour to allow the flavours to meld.

Peel and segment the grapefruit. Toss the kale with the rest of the dressing and arrange on four plates. Scatter with the sliced radishes. Pile the dressed beetroot on top, and decorate with the grapefruit segments.

Serves 4   Time taken: 1½ hours, including 1 hour standing

Per serving
Calories 194kcals; Protein 2g; Carbohydrates 16g; Dietary Fibre 3g; Sugar – Total 11g; Fat – Total 14g; Saturated Fat 2g; Vitamin C 74mg; Magnesium 27mg

Kale is a fantastic source of minerals, beta-carotene and folic acid, and this puts it firmly on my list of superfoods.

SPINACH SALAD WITH GARLIC YOGHURT DRESSING

Protein 16%
Carbohydrate 31%
Fat 53%

GI: very low
GL: very low

This is a good way to use the larger spinach leaves. Baby spinach leaves don't need much jazzing up, but the larger leaves, with their strong flavour and more robust texture, take kindly to a creamy dressing.

450 g	Fresh spinach	1 lb
2	Tomatoes, peeled and sliced	2
6	Spring onions, thinly sliced on the diagonal	6
5 tbsp	Natural live yoghurt	5 tbsp
2 tbsp	Extra virgin olive oil	2 tbsp
2	Garlic cloves, peeled and finely chopped	2
1 tbsp	Fresh oregano leaves	1 tbsp
	Sea salt and freshly ground black pepper	

Wash the spinach well in several changes of water. Dry the leaves carefully and tear into bite-sized pieces if necessary. Place in a salad bowl together with the tomatoes and spring onions.

Whisk together the yoghurt, olive oil, chopped garlic and oregano, and season to taste.

Toss the salad with the dressing and serve.

Serves 4   **Time taken: 15 minutes**

Per serving
Calories 124kcals; Protein 5g; Carbohydrates 11g; Dietary Fibre 4g; Sugar – Total 3g; Fat – Total 8g; Saturated Fat 1g; Vitamin C 49mg; Magnesium 101mg

Spinach is an excellent source of magnesium, needed by people with diabetes, because magnesium can help promote healthy insulin production. It can also reduce the craving for sweet foods that can contribute to the development of Type 2 diabetes.

DESSERTS

APPLE QUINOA PUDDING

Protein 10%
Carbohydrate 82%
Fat 8%

GI: medium
GL: medium

Quinoa is a good choice for a filling winter pudding, as it's high in protein and provides less starch than a wheat-based alternative. The yoghurt is important as the protein and fat it contains balance the carbohydrate and help to reduce the glycaemic load.

150 ml	Apple juice	¼ pint
150 ml	Water	¼ pint
110 g	Quinoa	4 oz
3 tbsp	Raisins	3 tbsp
½ tsp	Mixed spice	½ tsp
3	Dessert apples	3
2 tbsp	Organic molasses sugar	2 tbsp
Natural live yoghurt or soya yoghurt, to serve		

Place the apple juice, water, quinoa, raisins and mixed spice in a pan, and bring to the boil over medium heat, stirring. Lower the heat, cover and simmer for 15-20 minutes, or until the quinoa is tender and most of the liquid evaporated. Drain off and discard any liquid that is left.

Preheat the oven to 200°C/400°F/Gas Mark 6.

Spoon half the quinoa mixture into a 1.2 litre/2 pint ovenproof dish. Peel, core and slice the apples and arrange half the slices over the quinoa. Top with the remaining quinoa, and arrange the remaining apple slices on top. Sprinkle with the molasses sugar.

Bake for 25-30 minutes in the preheated oven, or until golden brown.

Serve with yoghurt.

Serves 4   **Time taken: 1 hour**

Per serving
Calories 233kcals; Protein 6g; Carbohydrates 51g; Dietary Fibre 4g; Sugar – Total 25g; Fat – Total 2g; Saturated Fat 0g; Vitamin C 6mg; Magnesium 88mg

Quinoa is a rich source of magnesium, a very important mineral for people with diabetes as it is needed for the synthesis of insulin. Molasses sugar is made from the part of the sugarcane left behind after the refining process. So although it is sugar, it is rich in minerals, especially iron.

APPLE AND PASSION FRUIT SNOW
WITH ALMOND WAFERS

Protein 9%   GI: medium
Carbohydrate 73%   GL: medium
Fat 18%

Apple snow was one of my favourite puddings from childhood, and here I have updated with the addition of passion fruit, which weren't available back then. Make sure the passion fruit are ripe – the skin should be wrinkled and hard.

	For the almond wafers:	
15 g	Unsalted butter, softened	½ oz
30 g	Organic raw cane sugar	1 oz
1	Organic, free range egg white	1
25 g	Plain or gluten-free flour	Scant 1 oz
1 tbsp	Flaked almonds	1 tbsp
	For the apple and passion fruit snow:	
450 g	Cooking apples	1 lb
3 tbsp	Concentrated apple juice	3 tbsp
3	Passion fruit	3
3	Organic, free range egg whites	3

Preheat the oven to 180°C/350°F/Gas Mark 4. Cover a large flat baking-tray with a sheet of non-stick baking parchment. Cream the butter and sugar until well mixed then beat in the egg whites followed by the flour.

Spoon a level dessertspoonful on to the baking tray and spread with the back of the spoon round and round into a flat circle. Sprinkle with the flaked nuts.

Repeat three more times so you have four tuiles on the sheet. Bake for 8-10 minutes until the edges turn light brown and the centres are pale golden. Remove from the oven, wait a few seconds then slide off with a palette knife on to a rack to cool. Repeat with the rest of the mixture. You should have 8 tuiles.

For the apple and passion fruit snow, peel, core and roughly chop the apples and put them in a pan with the concentrated apple juice and 3 tbsp water. Bring to the boil, lower the heat and simmer gently, covered, until the apple has cooked down to a mush. This will take about 20 minutes. Remove from the heat and stir vigorously with a wooden spoon to break down any remaining pieces of apple.

Cut the passion fruit in half and spoon out the pulp. Add to the apple purée and mix thoroughly.

Put the egg whites in a bowl and whisk until they form soft peaks. Fold the egg whites into the apple-passion fruit mixture. Spoon the apple foam into individual glass dishes and serve cold, accompanied by the almond tuiles.

Serves 4   **Time taken: 1 hour**

Per serving
Calories 212kcals; Protein 5g; Carbohydrates 41g; Dietary Fibre 4g; Sugar – Total 31g; Fat – Total 4g; Saturated Fat 2g; Vitamin C 10mg; Magnesium 19mg

Note: Because this recipe contains uncooked egg whites, it should not be served to pregnant women.

Apples are an excellent choice for people with diabetes as their glycaemic index is low and they provide soluble fibre which slows down glycaemic response.

APRICOT AND TOFU CHEESECAKE

Protein 18%   GI: medium
Carbohydrate 45%   GL: low
Fat 37%

*Fresh apricots are tricky customers. They can be utterly delicious if
you catch them at the right moment, but so often they are picked
before they are ripe and never reach ripe perfection. You can use
well-drained apricots tinned in their own juice for this recipe if you
cannot find good fresh ones.*

	For the base:	
30 g	Butter	1 oz
2 tbsp	Apple juice	2 tbsp
110 g	Oat and almond muesli (see page 51)	4 oz
	For the filling:	
285 g	Silken tofu	10 oz
225 g	Natural live yoghurt or soya yoghurt, drained in a sieve overnight	8 oz
4 tbsp	Apple juice	4 tbsp
2 tsp	Agar agar powder (or 1½ tbsp agar agar flakes)	2 tsp
	For the topping:	
6	Fresh apricots, halved and stoned	6
2 tbsp	All-fruit apricot jam	2 tbsp

Preheat the oven to 180°C/350°F/Gas Mark 4.

For the base, process the muesli in a food processor until it
forms fine crumbs. Melt the butter and apple juice over gentle heat
and mix it with the ground muesli. Spread it in an oiled 23 cm/
9 inch flan tin with a removable base, and bake for 5 minutes.
Cool and chill while you make the filling.

Place the tofu and drained yoghurt in a food processor and
process until smooth. Put the apple juice and agar agar powder into
a small pan and cook until the agar agar has dissolved – about 5
minutes. If you are using the agar agar flakes, you will need to
cook a bit longer. Stir into the yoghurt and tofu mixture.

Spread this mixture on to the chilled base and refrigerate until
set.

Remove the flan ring and place on a serving plate. Arrange the
apricot halves on the cake. Mix the apricot jam with a

tablespoonful of warm water, and brush onto the apricots.
Serve chilled.

Serves 6   **Time taken: 30 minutes plus setting time**

Per serving
Calories 210kcals; Protein 10g; Carbohydrates 25g; Dietary
Fibre 2g; Sugar – Total 10g; Fat – Total 9g; Saturated Fat 4g;
Vitamin C 4mg; Magnesium 34mg

Apricots are a useful source of beta-carotene, a good
antioxidant protective against free radical damage. They taste
sweet but provide relatively few calories. They also supply fibre
and have a low glycaemic index, so they make an excellent
choice for people with diabetes and for those who need to lose
weight.

BAKED BLACKBERRY CHEESECAKE

Protein 32%   GI: low
Carbohydrate 49%   GL: low
Fat 19%

*I love blackberries, especially the fact that they are free. My husband
and I pick as many as possible during the season. I like them raw on
my cereal at breakfast, or just simply mixed with yoghurt, and
they're good, too, stewed lightly with apple for all sorts of pies and
puddings. This cheesecake is best made with fresh raw blackberries,
but frozen, thawed blackberries will do almost as well. Drained
blackberries canned in natural juice are a third choice.*

175 g	Cottage cheese	6 oz
150 g	Natural live yoghurt or soya yoghurt	5 oz
1 tbsp	Wholemeal or gluten-free flour	1 tbsp
2 tbsp	Organic raw cane sugar	2 tbsp
1	Organic, free range egg	1
1	Organic, free range egg white	1
1/2	Lemon, finely grated rind and juice	1/2
200 g	Fresh or thawed frozen blackberries	7 oz

Preheat the oven to 180°C/350°F/Gas Mark 4. Oil an 18 cm/7 inch
loose-bottomed round cake tin, and line with greaseproof paper.
Place the cottage cheese in the food processor and process until

smooth, or rub through a wire sieve into a bowl. Add the yoghurt, flour, sugar, whole egg and egg white, mixing well. Then stir in the lemon rind and juice and the blackberries, reserving a few for garnish.

Spoon the mixture into the prepared cake tin and bake for 30-35 minutes, or until set. Turn off the oven and leave the cheesecake in the oven for another 30 minutes.

Take the cheesecake out of the oven, run a knife around the perimeter, then turn it out of the tin. Remove the greaseproof paper and leave to cool.

Serve the cheesecake at room temperature, sliced into sections and decorated with the reserved blackberries.

Serves 4   **Time taken: 1¼ hours**

Per serving
Calories 137kcals; Protein 11g; Carbohydrates 18g; Dietary Fibre 3g; Sugar – Total 6g; Fat – Total 3g; Saturated Fat 1g; Vitamin C 21mg; Magnesium 17mg

> I have used cottage cheese very little in this book, as dairy products (with the exception of live yoghurt) may be contraindicated for people with diabetes, particularly those with Type 1 diabetes. However, cottage cheese is a useful low-fat source of protein and can be included in the diet from time to time. If you are avoiding dairy products, you could substitute drained and mashed tofu for the cottage cheese.

BLUEBERRY AND LEMON YOGHURT

Protein 22%	GI: low
Carbohydrate 62%	GL: low
Fat 16%	

This is a beguilingly simple recipe but delicious. You need to use a thick yoghurt – I usually use a sheep's milk yoghurt such as that made by Woodlands Park Dairy in Dorset. If your yoghurt is a bit on the thin side, strain it in some clean muslin for a couple of hours to remove some of the whey before proceeding.

450 g	Natural live yoghurt	1 lb
150 g	Crème fraîche	5 oz
1 tbsp	Very finely grated lemon rind	1 tbsp
3 tbsp	Organic raw cane sugar	3 tbsp

Simply mix together the yoghurt, crème fraîche and lemon rind and sweeten to taste. Place most of the blueberries into four individual glass dishes, reserving a few for decoration, then spoon over the yoghurt mixture. Decorate with the remaining blueberries and serve chilled.

Serves 4   **Time taken: 10 minutes**

Per serving
Calories 120kcals; Protein 7g; Carbohydrates 20g; Dietary Fibre 2g; Sugar – Total 9g; Fat – Total 2g; Saturated Fat 1g; Vitamin C 9mg; Magnesium 3mg

Variations on this theme are endless and limited only to the fruit you have to hand. This dish is delicious with strawberries and exquisite with raspberries. Kiwi fruit, pears, fresh apricots or any other soft, sweet fruit would do very well too.

CHERRY BUCKWHEAT CRÊPES

Protein 11%	GI: medium
Carbohydrate 76%	GL: low
Fat 13%	

You could make these crêpes using only buckwheat flour, but without the addition of a lighter flour they can be a bit heavy and strong-tasting.

	For the crêpes:	
90 g	Buckwheat flour	3 oz
30 g	Unbleached white flour or gluten-free flour	1 oz
1	Large, organic free range egg	1
300 ml	Soya or rice milk mixed with water	½ pint
	For the filling:	
450 g	Black cherries, stoned	1 lb
3 tbsp	Concentrated apple juice	3 tbsp
1½ tsp	Arrowroot	1½ tsp

For the crêpes, put the flour, egg and milk and water mixture in the blender, and blend until well mixed. Leave the batter to rest while you make the filling.

For the filling, put the cherries and concentrated apple juice into a pan, bring to the boil over gentle heat, and simmer for 10–15 minutes or until the cherries are tender. Cool a little, then drain, reserving the syrup.

Now, make the crêpes. Heat a non-stick medium-sized frying pan and spray lightly with olive oil spray. Ladle in enough batter just to cover the base of the pan. Cook over medium-high heat until the surface bubbles and starts to dry. Turn and cook the other side until lightly browned, then slide the finished crêpe out onto kitchen paper and keep warm. Repeat with the remaining mixture. This should make 12 crêpes.

To finish the filling, mix about 2 tbsp of the syrup with the arrowroot in a small saucepan, then stir in the rest of the syrup. Heat gently, stirring, until the mixture boils, thickens and clears. Add the cherries and stir until heated through.

Spoon the cherries into the crêpes and fold into quarters. Serve hot with a spoonful of plain yoghurt.

Serves 6   **Time taken: 1 hour**

Per serving
Calories 173kals; Protein 5g; Carbohydrates 35g; Dietary Fibre 4g; Sugar – Total 18g; Fat – Total 3g; Saturated Fat 1g; Vitamin C 5mg; Magnesium 53mg

These crêpes incorporate two ingredients that are thought to be beneficial for people with diabetes – cherries and buckwheat. The contribution of cherries is their low GI, and buckwheat has been shown in several studies to help lower blood glucose.

CHERRY AND ALMOND CLAFOUTIS

Protein 12%   GI: medium
Carbohydrate 50%   GL: low
Fat 38%

A clafoutis is a French pudding consisting of fruit baked in a rich pancake batter. It's very easy, and delicious with apples, pears, apricots or blackberries. But it's best of all with cherries.

900 g	Cherries, washed and stoned	2 lb
2 tbsp	Brown rice flour or Doves Farm gluten-free flour	2 tbsp
4 tbsp	Maple syrup	4 tbsp

4	Organic free range eggs	4
60 g	Ground almonds	2 oz
225 ml	Soya or rice milk	½ pint
1 tbsp	Extra virgin olive oil	1 tbsp
2 tsp	Icing sugar (optional)	2 tsp
	Soya cream or yoghurt to serve	

Preheat the oven to 190°C/375°F/Gas Mark 5.

Oil a shallow baking dish. Put the cherries in the dish. Beat together the flour, maple syrup, eggs, ground almonds, soya or rice milk and olive oil (this is easiest done in a blender). Pour the batter over the cherries, and bake in the oven for 45 minutes, or until the clafoutis is puffed up and golden. To test whether it is cooked, insert a sharp knife or skewer into the middle – it should come out clean. If it doesn't, lower the heat to 150°C/300°F/Gas Mark 2 and continue cooking for another 10 minutes or so.

Serve dusted with icing sugar if liked, and with soya cream or yoghurt on the side.

Serves 6   **Time taken: 1 hour**

Per serving
Calories 299kcals; Protein 10g; Carbohydrates 39g; Dietary Fibre 5g; Sugar – Total 30g; Fat – Total 13g; Saturated Fat 2g; Vitamin C 10mg; Magnesium 64mg

Cherries are a rich source of copper, a deficiency of which may be a cause of osteoporosis. Certainly, it is known that a severe copper deficiency produces abnormalities in bone growth, which would imply that it is wise to make sure we get enough copper from our diet.

CINNAMON APPLE YOGHURT CAKE

Protein 5%   GI: medium
Carbohydrate 36%   GL: low
Fat 59%

This cake is based on a recipe by Donna Hay, the gifted and innovative Australian cookery writer. Her version, using sour cream, is richer and more indulgent than my pared-down version. Don't be put off by the amount of butter and sugar – the cake serves 8 people, so each serving contains only a small amount.

110 g	Butter	4 oz
4 tbsp	Suma pear and apple spread	4 tbsp
2 tsp	Cinnamon	2 tsp
2	Organic, free range eggs	2
150 g	Natural live yoghurt, drained of whey	5 oz
1 tbsp	Lemon juice	1 tbsp
225 g	Doves Farm gluten-free flour	8 oz
1 tsp	Baking powder	1 tsp
	For the topping:	
3 tbsp	Doves Farm gluten-free flour	3 tbsp
3 tbsp	Organic raw cane sugar	3 tbsp
3 tbsp	Ground pumpkin seeds	3 tbsp
1 tsp	Cinnamon	1 tsp
3	Green dessert apples, peeled, cored and thinly sliced	3

Preheat the oven to 180°C/350°F/Gas Mark 4. Grease a 23 cm/ 9 inch round springform cake tin.

Beat together the butter, concentrated apple juice and cinnamon, either by hand or with an electric mixer. Add the eggs and beat well. Fold in the drained yoghurt and lemon juice. Sift together the flour and baking powder and fold gently into the mixture. Spoon into the prepared cake tin.

For the topping, mix together the flour, sugar, ground pumpkin seeds and cinnamon, then toss the apple slices in this mixture. Arrange the apple slices over the top of the cake and sprinkle with any remaining topping. Bake for 1 hour or until a skewer inserted in the cake comes out clean. Serve warm or at room temperature with extra yoghurt if desired.

Variations: Try substituting pears, plums or apricots for the apples. Ground almonds or walnuts would work well instead of ground pumpkin seeds for the topping.

Serves 8 **Time taken: 1¹/₄ hours**

Per serving
Calories 307kcals; Protein 5g; Carbohydrates 43g; Dietary Fibre 2g; Sugar – Total 9g; Fat – Total 15g; Saturated Fat 8g; Vitamin C 3mg; Magnesium 29mg

CINNAMON CLEMENTINES

Protein 6% GI: medium
Carbohydrate 80% GL: medium-high
Fat 14%

This is a dessert I make at Christmas as an alternative to the ubiquitous Christmas pudding, which is too heavy to eat after the turkey and all the trimmings, disliked by many people and anyway pretty much out-of-bounds for people with diabetes. This is a light but festive alternative with the added benefit of blood-sugar-lowering cinnamon.

8	Clementines	8
300 ml	Apple juice	¹/₂ pint
2	Cinnamon sticks	2
2 tbsp	Cointreau or Grand Marnier (optional)	2 tbsp
2 tbsp	Shelled, unsalted pistachio nuts	2 tbsp

Using a vegetable peeler, pare the rind from two of the clementines, being careful not to include any pith, and cut into fine strips. Set aside.

Peel the clementines, removing every scrap of pith but keeping each fruit whole. Place in a heatproof bowl.

Place the apple juice, reserved peel and cinnamon sticks into a pan, bring to the boil and cook until reduced by half. Stir in the liqueur if using. Leave the syrup to cool for about 10 minutes, then pour over the clementines in the bowl. Cool, cover and chill overnight.

Before serving, skin the pistachios: cover them with boiling water for a few minutes. Drain and slip off the skins while still warm. Chop roughly and scatter over the clementines before serving. Serve with natural yoghurt.

Serves 4   **Time taken: 35 minutes**

Per serving
Calories 123kcals; Protein 2g; Carbohydrates 27g; Dietary Fibre 4g; Sugar – Total 22g; Fat – Total 2g; Saturated Fat 0g; Vitamin C 44mg; Magnesium 24mg

I make no apology for including so many recipes featuring cinnamon. There has been a lot of research into the benefits of cinnamon in the management of diabetes (see page 35) that consuming half a teaspoon per day seems like an excellent strategy. Although this doesn't sound like a large quantity, it may be quite difficult to use this much and you will be looking for innovative ways to include cinnamon in your diet. These clementines are just one idea.

FLOATING ISLANDS WITH PLUM SAUCE

Protein 8%   GI: medium
Carbohydrate 87%   GL: medium
Fat 5%

450 g	Plums	1 lb
300 ml	Apple juice	½ pint
2	Organic, free range egg whites	2
2 tbsp	Organic raw cane sugar	2 tbsp
	Fresh nutmeg, grated	

Halve and stone the plums. Place in a pan with the apple juice.
Bring to the boil, lower the heat, cover and simmer for 15-20
minutes or until the plums are tender. Cool and purée in a
liquidiser or food processor. Pour the resulting purée into a wide
sauté pan or frying pan and leave to simmer over a very gentle
heat.

For the 'islands', whisk the egg whites until they hold soft peaks.
Gradually whisk in the sugar, and continue whisking until the
meringue is stiff.

Using two tablespoons, form the meringue mixture into 8 oval
shapes and place into the simmering plum sauce. Cover and
simmer gently for 2-3 minutes, until the meringues are just set.
Serve hot with a sprinkling of fresh nutmeg.

Serves 4   **Time taken: 45 minutes**

Per serving
**Calories 135kcals; Protein 3g; Carbohydrates 31g; Dietary Fibre
2g; Sugar – Total 27g; Fat – Total 1g; Saturated Fat 0g; Vitamin
C 11mg; Magnesium 12mg**

The protein in the egg whites helps to mitigate the blood-sugar
raising effect of the sweet plums.

POACHED PEARS IN GINGER YOGHURT SAUCE

Protein 5%   GI: medium
Carbohydrate 88%   GL: medium
Fat 7%

Pears and ginger make a delicious combination.

4	Large dessert pears, such as Comice or Williams	4
1 tbsp	Lemon juice	1 tbsp
225 ml	Apple juice	8 fl oz
	Thinly pared rind of one lemon	
2	Pieces of stem ginger, chopped	2
2 tbsp	Syrup from the jar of ginger	2 tbsp
1/2 tsp	Arrowroot	1/2 tsp
100 g	Natural live yoghurt	3 1/2 oz

Preheat the oven to 180°C/350°F/Gas Mark 4.

Peel the pears thinly, leaving them whole with their stalks on. Brush with lemon juice to prevent discoloration. Using an apple corer or potato peeler, scoop out as much of the core as you can from the base of each pear.

Place the pears in an ovenproof dish together with apple juice and lemon rind. Cook in the preheated oven until tender – about half an hour – turning the pears from time to time so that they cook evenly.

Remove the pears to a plate to cool and pour the syrup into a pan. Bring to the boil and cook, uncovered, until reduced by half. Add the ginger and ginger syrup. Take out a spoonful or two of liquid and blend in a cup with the arrowroot, then return to the pan and mix well. Cook gently, stirring, until the mixture thickens and clears. This will only take a minute or two, then remove from the heat. Up to now the recipe can be made in advance.

Just before serving, mix the ginger syrup with the yoghurt and use to cover the base of four individual plates. Then slice the pears almost all the way through from base to stem, leaving the slices attached at the stem end. Finally, fan out the pears on the yoghurt and ginger sauce.

Serves 4   **Time taken: 1 hour**

Per serving
Calories 180kcals; Protein 2g; Carbohydrates 43g; Dietary Fibre 4g; Sugar – Total 37g; Fat – Total 1g; Saturated Fat 0g; Vitamin

C 12mg; Magnesium 14mg

> Arrowroot is a white powder extracted from the root of a West Indian plant. The native people, the Arawaks, used the substance to draw out toxins from people wounded by poison arrows – hence the name Arrowroot. It is used today as a thickener, usually for sweet sauces. It thickens at a lower temperature than cornflour, but cooking for more than a minute or two will cause the liquid to go thin again, so it should only be added at the end of cooking. Cornflour can be substituted but use a bit less.

PRUNE AND ORANGE CREAMS

Protein 9%
Carbohydrate 85%
Fat 6%

GI: medium
GL: low

This is very quick to make and uses ingredients you will probably already have to hand.

225 g	Ready to eat prunes or soaked dried prunes, roughly chopped	8 oz
150 ml	Orange juice	1/4 pint
225 g	Natural live yoghurt or soya yoghurt	8 oz
2 tbsp	Cointreau, Grand Marnier or brandy (optional)	2 tbsp
	The rind of half an orange, thinly pared and sliced into tiny matchsticks, to garnish	

Place the chopped prunes in a pan with the orange juice and bring to the boil over a gentle heat. Cover and simmer for about 5 minutes, until the prunes are tender and the liquid is reduced by half. Remove from the heat and allow to cool, then blend to a purée in the blender or food processor.

Stir the yoghurt, prune purée and liqueur (if using) lightly together to achieve a marbled effect. Spoon into individual glass dishes and garnish with the shreds of orange peel. Serve chilled.

Serves 4   **Time taken: 20 minutes**

Per serving
Calories 211kcals; Protein 5g; Carbohydrates 49g; Dietary Fibre

5g; Sugar – Total 7g; Fat – Total 1g; Saturated Fat 1g; Vitamin C 24mg; Magnesium 27mg

> Prunes have many virtues, not least their laxative effect. They do this by providing fibre for the good bacteria. These bacteria then ferment the fibre and in the process increase the bulk of the stools, which helps to relieve constipation. Prunes are also an excellent source of potassium which helps to maintain fluid balance and therefore good blood pressure levels.

RASPBERRIES AND PASSION FRUIT WITH COCONUT CUSTARD

Protein 7%
Carbohydrate 31%
Fat 62%

GI: low
GL: low

Passion fruit gives this pudding an exotic taste. As a variation, try it with pears, strawberries or blueberries instead of the raspberries.

300 g	Fresh raspberries	10 oz
2	Passion fruit	2
2 tbsp	Organic raw cane sugar	2 tbsp
	Coconut Custard:	
300 ml	Soya or rice milk, or goat's milk	1/2 pint
300 ml	Coconut milk	1/2 pint
1	Cinnamon stick	1
1/4 tsp	Freshly grated nutmeg	1/4 tsp
4	Cardamom pods, crushed	4
11/2 tbsp	Arrowroot	11/2 tbsp
	4 raspberries and 4 sprigs of mint, to serve	

Using a fork, mash the raspberries in a small bowl until the juice runs.

Halve the passion fruit, scoop out the seeds and put these in a separate bowl.

For the custard, put all but 3 tbsp of the milk into a pan, add the cinnamon, nutmeg and crushed cardamom and bring to just below boiling point over a gentle heat. Remove from the heat, cover and leave to infuse for 30 minutes. Strain through a sieve and discard the cinnamon and crushed cardamom.

Blend the arrowroot with the reserved 3 tbsp milk and stir in the warm milk. Heat gently, stirring until boiling, then simmer, stirring constantly, for 1-2 minutes or until thickened. Leave to cool to room temperature.

Add the passion fruit pulp to the coconut custard and stir in sugar to taste, using as little as possible.

Place alternate spoonfuls of raspberry pulp and the coconut custard mixture into individual glass dishes. Stir lightly to create a swirled effect, and decorate each serving with a whole raspberry and a sprig of fresh mint. Serve chilled.

Serves 4   **Time taken: 1 hour**

Per serving
Calories 233kcals; Protein 5g; Carbohydrates 19g; Dietary Fibre 8g; Sugar – Total 8g; Fat – Total 17g; Saturated Fat 14g; Vitamin C 22mg; Magnesium 64mg

Coconut milk has the same virtues as coconut oil, but in lesser proportion as it is only 24% fat.

BASICS

STOCK

The essence of a good soup is the stock you use to make it.
There are one or two good organic stocks on the market, such as
Marigold or Kallo, but nothing beats making your own. It should
be a habit always to have some stock on hand in the fridge, but if
there's simply no room, or you've got more stock than you know
what to do with, you can make stock cubes to freeze. When you
have made your stock, boil it hard until it is reduced to a fraction
of its original volume, then freeze the resultant concentrated stock
in ice cube trays. These 'stock cubes' can then be diluted with
water to make instant home-made stock.

VEGETABLE STOCK

1	Large onion	1
2	Large carrots	2
3	Sticks of celery	3
4	Outside leaves of lettuce	4
	Potato peelings	
	Parsley stalks	
1	Bay leaf	1
6	Peppercorns	6
1½ litres	Water	2½ pints

Simmer all the ingredients together for about half an hour.
Drain and use as directed in soups and sauces. Since it is so quick
to make I don't usually bother to keep vegetable stock on hand,
but it should keep for up to a week in the fridge or four months in
the freezer.
Makes about 1 litre/1³/₄ pints

Per litre
**Calories 268kcal; Protein 9g; Carbohydrates 61g; Sugar – Total
15g; Dietary Fibre 13g; Fat – Total 1g; Saturated Fat 0g; Vitamin
C 107mg; Magnesium 175mg**

CHICKEN STOCK

The longer and slower you can cook your stock the better. A slow cooker is ideal – if you have one of these, put it on low all night. If you have an Aga, put it in a covered ovenproof dish and cook in the slow oven for several hours.

1	Cooked chicken carcase	1
1	Large onion, peeled and roughly chopped	1
2	Large carrots, roughly chopped	2
3	Sticks of celery, roughly chopped	3
	Parsley stalks	
1	Bay leaf	1
6	Peppercorns	6
1/2 tsp	Sea salt	1/2 tsp
11/2 litres	Water	21/2 pints

Put all the ingredients in a large pan and bring to the boil. Cover and simmer over very low heat for 1-2 hours. The slower you cook it, the more goodness will be extracted, and the clearer your stock will be. If you boil it too hard it will go cloudy.

Drain in a sieve or colander. If you are using the stock straight away, skim off and discard any fat. If not, cool the stock completely before skimming the fat (it will be easier to remove when cool). It will keep for up to three days in the fridge or for three months in the freezer.

Makes about 1 litre/1³/₄ pints

Per litre
Calories 353kcal; Protein 13g; Carbohydrates 69g; Dietary Fibre 17g; Sugar – Total 20g; Fat – Total 3g; Saturated Fat 0g; Vitamin C 117mg; Magnesium 167mg

FISH STOCK

2 tbsp	Extra virgin olive oil	2 tbsp
1	Onion, roughly chopped	1
2	Carrots, chopped	2
2 sticks	Celery, chopped	2 sticks
675 g	Bones and trimmings of any white fish such as cod, haddock, whiting or plaice	1½ lb
1½ litres	Water	2½ pints
1 tbsp	White wine vinegar	1 tbsp
3	Whole black peppercorns	3
½ tsp	Sea salt	½ tsp

Heat the oil in a heavy pot over moderately high heat until hot but not smoking, then sauté the onion, carrots, and celery, stirring occasionally, until golden. Add the fish bones and trimmings, water, vinegar, peppercorns, and salt. Bring to the boil, skim the froth, then reduce heat and simmer, uncovered, for 30 minutes.

Pour the stock through a fine-mesh sieve into a large bowl. If you are using the stock straight away, skim off and discard any fat. If not, cool the stock completely before skimming the fat (it will be easier to remove when cool). It will keep for a week in the fridge.

Makes about 1 litre/1¾ pints

Per litre
Calories 170kcal; Protein 23g; Carbohydrates 0g; Dietary Fibre 0g; Sugar – Total 0g; Fat – Total 8g; Saturated Fat 2g; Vitamin C 1mg; Magnesium 70mg

SAUCES AND SALAD DRESSINGS

BASIC TOMATO SAUCE

1 tbsp	Extra virgin olive oil	1 tbsp
1	Medium onion, peeled and finely chopped	1
1	Carrot, finely chopped	1
1	Stick celery, finely chopped	1
2	Garlic cloves, peeled and finely chopped	2
4 tbsp	Red or white wine	4 tbsp
900 g	Fresh tomatoes, peeled and chopped, or 2 x 400 g cans of chopped Italian tomatoes	2 lb
	Bouquet garni of 1 bay leaf, 1 sprig each of parsley, thyme and rosemary	
	Sea salt and freshly ground black pepper	

Heat the oil over medium heat, and sauté the onion, carrot, celery and garlic until soft but not browned. Add the wine, tomatoes, bouquet garni and seasoning. Bring to the boil, reduce the heat to low, cover and simmer for one hour, stirring from time to time. Remove the bouquet garni, cool and purée in the food processor. Keep refrigerated and use within four days or freeze for future use.
Makes 1 litre/1³/4 pints – approx. 12 servings

Per serving
Calories 81kcals; Protein 2g; Carbohydrates 12g; Dietary Fibre 2g; Sugar – Total 6g; Fat – Total 3g; Saturated Fat 1g; Vitamin C 15mg; Magnesium 14mg

BASIC VINAIGRETTE

Whisk together 4 tablespoons cold pressed extra virgin olive oil, 1 tablespoon flax oil and 1 tablespoon cider vinegar, wine vinegar or lemon juice. Season with sea salt, freshly ground black pepper and a little dry mustard powder to taste.

Variations: Substitute walnut oil, hazelnut oil or avocado oil for the olive oil.

SOYA MAYONNAISE

Using a blender, combine 90 g/3 oz silken tofu, 1 tablespoon cider vinegar, 1 tablespoon concentrated apple juice and seasoning to taste. With the machine running, add 6 tablespoons extra virgin olive oil, drop by drop at first, and then in a steady stream, as for mayonnaise. Add a crushed clove or two of garlic for garlic mayonnaise.

MISO DRESSING

Simply blend together 4 parts basic vinaigrette, 2 parts soya mayonnaise and 1 part miso. This dressing is delicious on grated root vegetables.

GAZPACHO DRESSING

This is a deliciously appetising dressing which enhances the look and flavour of different lettuces. The proportions are variable according to what you have available.

1	Garlic clove	1
1/2	Fresh green chilli	1/2
1/2	Small cucumber	1/2
1/2	Red pepper	1/2
3	Spring onions	3
150 ml	Extra virgin olive oil	1/4 pint
1 tbsp	Cider vinegar	1 tbsp
1 tbsp	Fresh lemon juice	1 tbsp
1 tbsp	Fresh basil, chopped	1 tbsp
	Freshly ground black pepper	

Whiz all the ingredients in the liquidiser and keep in the fridge. Shake well and drizzle over salad, vegetables or rice.

SUNFLOWER OR PUMPKIN SPREAD

Butter has its uses in cooking – being a saturated fat it is stable at high temperatures, and it adds a rich flavour to foods. However, there are many healthier and more nutritious spreads on the market. Try nut butters such as almond or cashew nut butter, or my latest favourite, Meridian's brazil nut butter (see Useful Addresses). For those who cannot tolerate nuts but would like a spread full of essential fatty acids and minerals, try using seeds instead.

110 g	Sunflower or pumpkin seeds	4 oz
1-2 tbsp	Organic, cold-pressed sunflower or pumpkin seed oil	1-2 tbsp
	Sea salt and freshly ground black pepper	
1 tbsp	Water or lemon juice	1 tbsp

Grind the seeds in an electric grinder until a fine powder is formed. Transfer to the food processor and, with the machine running, add half the oil. Gradually add the rest of the oil, if necessary, until the desired consistency is reached. Season to taste and stir in the water or lemon juice – this helps to emulsify the mixture. Home-made nut or seed butter is chunkier than the commercial variety because a domestic blender cannot grind as finely. Keep refrigerated and use within 3-4 days.
Makes 8 servings

Per serving
Calories 72kcals; Protein 3g; Carbohydrates 2g; Dietary Fibre 0g; Sugar – Total 0g; Fat – Total 6g; Saturated Fat 1g; Vitamin C 0mg; Magnesium 59mg

A word of caution about nuts, seeds and nut butters. Because of their highly unsaturated fat content, they are all prone to rancidity if not stored carefully. Always make or purchase in small quantities and keep them away from heat and light, preferably in the fridge. If you don't wish to make your own, Omega Nutrition make a delicious smooth pumpkin seed butter, available from Higher Nature (see Useful Addresses).

BARLEY BREAD

Protein 14%   GI: medium/high
Carbohydrate 82%   GL: medium
Fat 4%

Barley flour is low in gluten, so that a loaf made with all barley flour will be dense and heavy, and its earthy flavour is an acquired taste. However, I have found by experimenting that using about a ratio of 2:1 wheat and barley flour together with some soaked pearl barley results in a flavoursome loaf with a relatively low glycaemic index (for bread, that is). There is no fat in this loaf so it should be eaten fresh the day it is made, though it's fine for toast the next day.

100 g	Pearl barley (300 g/10$\frac{1}{2}$ oz cooked)	3$\frac{1}{2}$ oz
200 ml	Hand-hot water	$\frac{1}{3}$ pint
1 tsp	Runny honey	1 tsp
2 tsp	Active dry yeast	2 tsp
125 g	Organic strong white flour	4$\frac{1}{2}$ oz
110 g	Barley flour	4 oz
125 g	Organic stoneground wholemeal flour	4$\frac{1}{2}$ oz
1$\frac{1}{2}$ tsp	Sea salt	1$\frac{1}{2}$ tsp
1 tbsp	Organic barley flakes, for the topping	1 tbsp

First, cook the barley for about one hour, until nearly tender but still with some bite. Drain and cool.

Put half the water and the honey into a small bowl. Sprinkle in the yeast and leave in a warm place for 5 minutes. Stir to dissolve.

Mix the three flours and salt in a large bowl. Stir in the soaked and drained pearl barley. Pour in the yeast mixture and most of the rest of the water. Stir well to mix, then add the rest of the water as needed to make a sticky dough.

Turn out the dough onto a work surface sprinkled with barley flour. Knead until smooth. This will take at least 10 minutes.

Place the dough in an oiled bowl and cover with a tea towel. Leave in a warm place to rise until doubled in size, about 2 hours. Turn out and knead again to knock back the dough. Form into a loaf and place in an oiled 500 g/1 lb loaf tin. Cover again and leave to prove in a warm place until again doubled in size. The proving should be quicker this time – about 30-40 minutes.

Preheat the oven to 200°C/400°F/Gas Mark 6.

Brush the loaf with water and sprinkle on some barley flakes. Bake for one hour or until the loaf is golden and the base sounds

hollow when tapped. Turn out and cool on a wire rack.
Makes 1 loaf, approximately 15 slices

Per slice
**Calories 106kcals; Protein 4g; Carbohydrates 23g; Dietary Fibre
4g; Sugar – Total 1g; Fat – Total 1g; Saturated Fat 0g; Vitamin C
0mg; Magnesium 6mg**

This bread can also be made successfully in a bread machine,
using instant yeast and no honey. I use the wholewheat
programme on my machine and this quantity makes an extra
large loaf. As I am lucky enough to live very close to Bacheldre
Watermill, I use their wonderful organic stoneground flour for
all my baking (see Useful Addresses).

RYE CRISPBREAD

Protein 18%
Carbohydrate 71%
Fat 11%

GI: medium
GL: medium

This is based on a Swedish recipe for Knäckebröd, which are round fat-free crispbreads, usually made with whole rye grain and wheat flour. Knäckebröd is normally baked at a very high temperature for a short time and then left until thoroughly dry before storing. In Sweden crispbread is often used as a basis for Smørrebrød – Swedish open sandwiches.

350 g	Organic whole rye flour	12 oz
110 g	Organic rye flakes	4 oz
1 tsp	Instant yeast	1 tsp
2 tbsp	Sesame seed	2 tbsp
1 tsp	Sea salt	1 tsp
300 ml	Hand-hot water	½ pint

Place the flour, rye flakes, yeast, sesame seed and salt in a bowl. Stir in the water until a stiff dough is formed, then turn out onto a floured surface and knead well. Rye dough is hard to knead, but persevere until the dough feels smooth and no longer sticky. Place in an oiled bowl and leave in a warm place until the dough has risen slightly – about one hour.

Turn out the dough and knead again. Roll out as thinly as possible and cut into rectangles or discs. Place these on oiled baking trays and poke holes in the crispbreads with a knitting needle or fork. Cover with a cloth and leave to rise in a warm place for half an hour.

Preheat the oven to its highest setting: 230°C/450°F/Gas Mark 8.

Bake the crispbreads for 3-4 minutes, then turn over and bake the other side for a further 2-3 minutes.

Cool on a wire rack and store in an airtight tin.

Makes 24 crispbreads

Per slice
Calories 69kcals; Protein 3g; Carbohydrates 13g; Dietary Fibre 3g; Sugar – Total 0g; Fat – Total 1g; Saturated Fat 0g; Vitamin C 0mg; Magnesium 3mg

MENU PLANNER

In devising these menus I have aimed for a low ratio of carbohydrate to protein and a low glycaemic load over each day.

	Breakfast	Lunch	Evening Meal	Macro-nutrient Ratio (protein:carb:fat)
Week 1				
Monday	Apple, pear and tofu smoothie	White bean and mint hummus with raw vegetables	Grilled sardines with vegetable linguine Broccoli with garlic	20:35:45
Tuesday	Chickpea and tomato frittata	Two-lentil soup with coriander Fresh fruit	Tofu fajitas Mixed vegetables	20:40:40
Wednesday	Baked eggs with mushrooms	Two-lentil soup with coriander Rye toast	Grilled chicken with quinoa and lemons Steamed vegetables	25:29:46
Thursday	Poached egg with grilled tomatoes Wholegrain and seed muffins	Cold chicken with avocado, grapefruit and alfalfa salad	Puy lentils with olives and anchovies Blueberry and lemon yoghurt	19:38:43
Friday	Apricot, soya and plum smoothie	White bean and mint hummus with crudités and oatcakes	Trout fillets with lettuce and fennel Quinoa pilaff with green leaves	18:46:36
Saturday	Rainbow fruit salad with natural live yoghurt and 1 tbsp ground seeds	Broccoli soup with horseradish Barley bread with quick sardine pâté	Avocado, grapefruit and alfalfa salad Grilled mackerel Butter beans with fennel	15:40:45
	Boiled egg and barley bread toast	Butter bean with parsley pesto Bean and seed sprouts with avocado dressing	Cinnamon smoked duck Stir-fried vegetables Apple and passion fruit snow with Almond wafers	21:51:28

	Breakfast	Lunch	Evening Meal	Macro-nutrient Ratio (protein:carb:fat)
Week 2				
Monday	Oat porridge with grated apple and ground seeds	Cream of avocado soup with coconut milk	Turkey with fennel and cashew cream Steamed vegetables	15:42:43
Tuesday	Baked beans on rye toast	Cold chicken with large mixed salad	Buckwheat pancakes with ratatouille	30:47:23
Wednesday	Buckwheat pancakes with fresh fruit	Scotch eggs with a difference Mixed salad	Grilled trout with salsa verde Broccoli with garlic	18:42:40
Thursday	Chickpea and tomato frittata	Gazpacho with aubergine croûtons	Soya bean and mango chutney casserole Braised kale	15:36:49
Friday	Oat and almond muesli with natural live yoghurt	Soya bean and mango chutney casserole Chinese-style broccoli salad	Thai-style salmon fishcakes with cucumber salad Stir-fried bean sprouts	24:32:44
Saturday	Rainbow fruit salad with natural live yoghurt and 1 tbsp ground seeds	Omelette with salad	Buckwheat noodles with tofu, tahini sauce and vegetables	23:40:37
Sunday	Raspberry muesli sundae	Roast guinea fowl with walnut sauce Baked blackberry cheesecake	Butter beans with fennel	23:51:26
Week 3				
Monday	Yoghurt cheese with apricots and walnuts	June's spicy chana dal soup	Roasted mackerel with horseradish cream Warm East-West salad	18:45:37

	Breakfast	Lunch	Evening Meal	Macro-nutrient Ratio (protein:carb:fat)
Tuesday	Apricot, soya and plum smoothie	Cold roasted mackerel with mixed salad	Amaranth and lentil cakes Moghlai spinach	18:37:45
Wednesday	Marion's breakfast	Fennel and red cabbage salad with pumpkin seeds	Turkey with fennel and cashew cream Steamed vegetables	25:47:28
Thursday	Oat and almond muesli with natural live yoghurt and seeds	Two-lentil soup with coriander	Scotch eggs with a difference Fennel and red cabbage salad with pumpkin seeds	18:48:34
Friday	Baked eggs with mushrooms	Scotch eggs with a difference Green salad	Two-lentil soup with coriander Thai-style salmon fishcakes with cucumber salad	20:42:38
Saturday	Tropical tofu smoothie	Cold poached salmon Greek whole mushroom salad, green salad	Chana dal with coconut and spices Brown rice and barley Cinnamon jelly with roasted plums	21:47:32
Sunday	Oat and almond muesli with yoghurt and fruit	Grilled sardines with vegetable linguine	Cinnamon smoked duck Raspberries and passion fruit with coconut custard	20:24:56
Week 4				
Monday	Buckwheat pancakes with apple and almond filling	Cold smoked duck with mixed salad	Soya bean and mango chutney casserole	25:33:42
Tuesday	Oat and citrus smoothie	Spinach salad with garlic yoghurt dressing and soya beans	Salmon with minted pea purée and asparagus	29:35:36

	Breakfast	Lunch	Evening Meal	Macro-nutrient Ratio (protein:carb:fat)
Wednesday	Baked beans on rye toast	Cold salmon with lime-scented carrot and cucumber salad	Chilli tofu and coconut stew	28:30:42
Thursday	Tropical tofu smoothie	Quick sardine pâté on rye toast Fresh fruit	Black bean cakes with tomato and orange salsa	27:36:37
Friday	Chickpea and tomato frittata	Chana dal with spinach	Coconut fish curry Brown rice Green vegetable stir fry	22:44:34
Saturday	Apple, pear and tofu smoothie	Barley and spring vegetable risotto	Chilli mussels with garlic rye toast Warm East-West salad Prune and orange creams	20:48:32
Sunday	More than tomato juice Baked eggs with mushrooms	Crispy polenta with wild mushrooms and coriander pesto	Chicken in coconut milk Stir-fried green vegetables Cinnamon clementines	22:32:46

SHOPPING LIST

Vegetables, emphasise:
Beansprouts
Beetroot and beetroot greens (raw)
Broccoli
Cabbage
Celery
Chicory
Chinese cabbage
Courgettes
Garlic
Jerusalem artichokes
Kale
Mushrooms
Olives
Onions
Peppers
Radishes
Sea vegetables
Spinach
Sweet potatoes
Sweetcorn
Tomatoes

Fruits, emphasise:
Apples
Apricots, unsulphured dried or fresh
Avocados
Berry fruits
Cherries
Grapefruit
Grapes
Nectarines
Peaches
Pears
Plums

Note: treat cooked starchy root vegetables with caution owing to their high GI values (e.g. cooked parsnips, mashed potatoes)

Whole Grains
Amaranth
Brown rice
Buckwheat
Nature's Path cereals such as Mesa Sunrise, Millet Flakes etc
Organic oat flakes and oat groats
Pearl barley, pot barley
Polenta
Quinoa
Wholemeal pastas (any kind)

Protein Foods
Oily fish such as wild or organic salmon, mackerel, sea bass, herrings, trout, anchovies
White fish such as cod, haddock, plaice etc
Chicken, duck and guinea fowl (without skin)
Rabbit
Eggs, free range and organic
Lean meat, all visible fat removed
Combinations of pulses, whole grains and nuts/seeds

Flour
Barley flour
Brown rice flour
Buckwheat flour
Chickpea flour
Gluten-free flour such as Dove's Farm
Stone-ground organic wholemeal flour such as Bacheldre Mill

hazelnut,

Nuts and seeds, raw
Flax seed (linseed)
Pumpkin seed
Sesame seeds
Sunflower seeds
Almonds
Brazil nuts
Walnuts
Nut and seed butters (e.g. almond, tahini)

Pulses, any kind such as
Black beans
Butter beans
Chana dal
Chickpeas
Haricot beans
Kidney beans
Lentils, red, green and Puy
Soya beans and soya products such
   as tofu

Fats and Oils
Cold pressed extra virgin olive oil
Organic coconut oil
Butter in moderation
Flax seed oil, walnut oil, avocado oil,
   pumpkin seed oil for salads

Spices – include
Cinnamon
Fenugreek seed
Ginger
Juniper berries

Beverage Options
Herbal teas
Ginseng tea
Dandelion coffee
Green tea
Carob with soya, rice or nut milk

Sweeteners – minimal use only
Apple juice
Concentrated apple juice (Meridian)
Molasses
A little honey or maple syrup

Dairy products (if using)
Organic natural live yoghurt
Cottage cheese
Occasional use of Parmesan and goats/
   sheeps cheese

Optional milk alternatives
Soya milk
Rice Dream
Oat milk
Coconut milk

Bread alternatives
Rye bread (100% is best)
Rye crackers
Barley bread
Burgen Soya and Linseed bread (low GI)

Seasonings
Miso
Tamari/Shoyu (naturally brewed soy sauce)
Sea salt or low-sodium salt
Fresh herbs of all kinds

Convenience Foods
Tinned beans – any kind
Sardines or pilchards in olive oil
Tomatoes – tinned/paste/dried/salsa
Hummus
Falafel – Cauldron Foods
Covent Garden soups
Marinated tofu etc
Sugar free jams – Whole Earth

Food Equipment
Grinder – for nuts and seeds
Food processor
Juicer for vegetable juices
Pump-action spray for olive oil

THE GLYCAEMIC INDEX AND GLYCAEMIC LOAD

This is an extract of the latest tables available, which were published in 2002. Not all foods have been tested, and for reasons of space I have limited the extract here to more commonly used foods. The GI in these tables is based on an assumption that pure glucose has a GI of 100. Please note the following:

● A GI of 70 or more is high, a GI of 56 to 69 inclusive is medium, and a GI of 55 or less is low
● A GL of 20 or more is high, a GL of 11 to 19 inclusive is medium, and a GL of 10 or less is low
● Look for carbohydrate foods that are both low GI *and* low GL.

Food	GI Glucose	GL
BAKERY PRODUCTS		
Sponge cake, plain	46	16.6
Croissant	67	17.5
Crumpet	69	13.1
Doughnut	76	17.4
Pastry	59	15.4
BEVERAGES		
Cola soft drink	53	13.9
Orange soft drink	68	22.8
Sparkling glucose drink	95	39.7
Lemon squash soft drink	58	17.0
Apple juice, mean of three studies	40	11.7
Carrot juice, freshly made	43	10.0
Cranberry juice drink	56	16.4
Grapefruit juice, unsweetened	48	10.7
Orange juice, mean of two studies	50	12.8
Pineapple juice, unsweetened	46	15.6
Tomato juice, canned	38	3.5
BREADS		
Baguette, white, plain	95	14.7
Barley kernel bread, mean of two studies	46	9.4
Hamburger bun	61	9.2
Gluten-free white bread, sliced (gluten-free wheat starch)	80	11.9
Wholegrain pumpernickel	46	5.2
Wholemeal rye bread, mean of four studies	58	8.4
White bread, mean of six studies	70	9.7
White bread with butter	59	28.5
Wholemeal bread, mean of thirteen studies	71	9.5
Soya and linseed loaf	36	3.2
Pita bread, white	57	9.5
BREAKFAST CEREALS		
All-Bran™ (Kellogg's)	38	8.7
Bran Flakes™ (Kellogg's)	74	13.2
Cornflakes, mean of five studies	81	20.8
Natural muesli, mean of two studies	49	9.6
Muesli, toasted	43	7.1
Nutrigrain™ (Kellogg's)	66	9.9
Porridge made from rolled oats, mean of eight studies	58	12.8

Food	GI Glucose	GL
Puffed Wheat (Quaker Oats Co)	67	13.5
Raisin Bran™ (Kellogg's)	61	11.7
Rice Krispies™ (Kellogg's)	82	21.0
Shredded Wheat™ (Nabisco Brands Ltd)	83	16.6
Special K™ (Kellogg's)	54	11.3
Sultana Bran™ (Kellogg's)	73	13.7
Weetabix, mean of seven studies	70	13.0
CEREAL GRAINS		
Amaranth eaten with milk and non-nutritive sweetener	97	21.0
Pearl barley, mean of five studies	25	10.6
Buckwheat, mean of three studies	54	16.1
Corn tortilla	52	12.4
Cornmeal (polenta), mean of two studies	69	9.0
Couscous, mean of two studies	65	22.7
Millet, boiled	71	25.2
Arborio, risotto rice, boiled	69	36.2
Boiled white rice, mean of 12 studies	64	23.3
Boiled long grain rice, mean of 10 studies	56	22.9
Glutinous rice, white, cooked in rice cooker	98	31.0
Jasmine rice, white long grain, cooked in rice cooker	109	46.1
Basmati rice, white, boiled	58	21.8
Brown rice, mean of three studies	55	17.9
Rye, whole kernels, mean of three studies	34	12.9
Wheat, whole kernels, mean of four studies	41	14.0
Wheat tortilla (Mexican)	30	7.8
Bulgur wheat, mean of four studies	48	12.4
BISCUITS AND CRACKERS		
Digestive biscuits, mean of three studies	59	9.7
Rich Tea biscuits	55	10.4
Shortbread	64	9.9
Rice cakes, mean of three studies	78	17.0
Ryvita, mean of four studies	64	10.5
DAIRY PRODUCTS AND ALTERNATIVES		
Custard, home made from milk, wheat starch, and sugar	43	7.1
Ice cream, mean of five studies	61	7.9
Milk, full-fat, mean of five studies	27	3.1
Milk, skim	32	4.0
Milk, condensed, sweetened	61	17.0
Yoghurt	36	3.4
Low-fat, fruit yoghurt with aspartame	14	1.8
Soy milk, full-fat, 120 mg calcium	36	6.4
Soy yoghurt, peach and mango, 2% fat, sugar	50	13.0
FRUIT		
Apples, raw, mean of six studies	38	5.5
Apricots, raw	57	5.2
Apricots, canned in light syrup	64	12.0
Apricots, dried (Australia)	30	8.0
Banana, mean of 10 studies	52	12.4
Cherries, raw	22	2.7
Dates, dried	103	41.6
Figs, dried	61	15.7
Grapefruit, raw	25	2.7
Grapes, mean of two studies	46	8.2
Kiwi fruit, mean of two studies	53	6.2

Food	GI Glucose	GL
Lychee, canned in syrup and drained	79	16.1
Mango, mean of three studies	51	8.5
Oranges, mean of six studies	42	4.6
Papaya, mean of three studies	59	10.2
Peaches, mean of two studies	42	4.6
Peaches, canned, mean of two studies	38	4.2
Pears, raw, mean of four studies	38	4.2
Pineapple, mean of two studies	59	7.4
Plums, mean of two studies	39	4.8
Prunes	29	9.7
Raisins	64	28.5
Strawberries, fresh	40	1.3
Sultanas	56	25.2
Watermelon, raw	72	4.3

LEGUMES AND NUTS

Food	GI Glucose	GL
Baked beans, canned, mean of two studies	48	7.4
Black Beans	30	6.8
Blackeyed beans, boiled, mean of two studies	42	12.8
Butter beans, mean of three studies	31	6.1
Chickpeas, dried, boiled, mean of four studies	28	8.3
Haricot beans, mean of five studies	38	11.8
Kidney beans, mean of eight studies	28	6.9
Black beans, soaked overnight, cooked 45 min	20	4.9
Green lentils, mean of three studies	30	5.1
Red lentils, mean of four studies	26	4.8
Marrowfat peas, dried, boiled	47	
Mung beans, germinated	25	4.3
Peas, dried, boiled	22	1.9
Pinto beans, dried, boiled	39	10.0
Soya beans, dried, boiled, mean of two studies	18	1.1
Soya beans, canned	14	0.8
Split peas, yellow, boiled 20 min	32	6.1

CONVENIENCE FOODS AND MIXED MEALS

Food	GI Glucose	GL
Fish Fingers	38	7.3
Pizza, plain baked dough, served with parmesan cheese and tomato sauce	80	21.6
Sirloin chop with mixed vegetables and mashed potato, home made	66	34.9
Spaghetti bolognaise, home made	52	25.0
Stir-fried vegetables with chicken and boiled white rice, home made	73	54.7

PASTA AND NOODLES

Food	GI Glucose	GL
Corn pasta, gluten-free	78	32.4
Gluten-free pasta, maize starch, boiled 8 min	54	22.5
Rice noodles, dried, boiled	61	23.5
Rice noodles, freshly made, boiled	40	15.4
Rice pasta, brown, boiled 16 min	92	34.8
Rice and maize pasta, gluten-free	76	36.9
Soba noodles, instant, reheated in hot water, served with soup	46	22.3
White spaghetti, boiled, mean of three cooking times	57	27.3
Wholemeal spaghetti, boiled, mean of two studies	37	15.5
Split pea and soya pasta shells, gluten-free	29	8.9
Udon noodles, plain, reheated 5 min	62	30.0
Vermicelli, white, boiled	35	15.5

Food	GI Glucose	GL
SNACK FOODS AND CONFECTIONERY		
Chocolate, milk, mean of four studies	43	12.0
Mars Bar®	68	27.1
Cashew nuts, salted	22	2.8
Peanuts, mean of three studies	14	0.8
Popcorn, mean of two studies	72	7.7
Potato crisps, mean of two studies	54	11.4
Snickers Bar®	68	23.1
Twix® Cookie Bar, caramel	44	17.0
SOUPS		
Green Pea soup, canned	66	27.3
Lentil soup, canned	44	9.0
Minestrone soup	39	7.1
Tomato soup	38	6.4
SUGARS		
Honey, mean of 11 types	55	9.8
VEGETABLES		
Peas, mean of three studies	48	3.4
Pumpkin	75	3.3
Sweet corn, mean of six studies	54	9.3
Beetroot	64	4.6
Carrots, raw	16	1.2
Cooked carrots, mean of four studies	47	2.7
Parsnips	97	12.1
Baked potato, mean of four studies	85	25.6
Boiled potatoes, mean of five studies	50	13.9
Mashed potato, mean of three studies	74	14.5
New potato, mean of three studies	57	12.0
Sweet potato, mean of five studies	61	17.0
Swede	72	7.5

Source: Foster-Powell, et al, *International table of glycaemic index and glycaemic load values:* 2002, Am J Clin Nutr 2002; 76:5-56

USEFUL ADDRESSES

DIABETES-RELATED ORGANISATIONS
Diabetes UK
10 Parkway, London NW1 7AA
Tel: 020 7424 1000
Fax: 020 7424 1001
Email info@diabetes.org.uk
Website: www.diabetes.org.uk
The leading charity working with people with diabetes.

Diabetes Research & Wellness Foundation
101-102 Northney Marina, Hayling Island, Hampshire PO11 0NH
Tel: 023 9263 7808
Fax: 023 9263 6137
Website: www.diabeteswellnessnet.org.uk
A registered charity, finances research into diabetes and supports people with diabetes through the Diabetes Wellness Network.

Juvenile Diabetes Research Foundation
25 Gosfield Street, London W1W 6EB
Tel: 020 7436 3112
Fax: 020 7436 3039
Website: www.jdrf.org.uk
Founded in 1986 by families living with diabetes, with the aim of finding a cure and improving the lives of their children.

DIABETES-RELATED WEBSITES
www.mendosa.com
David Mendosa is a freelance medical writer and consultant specialising in diabetes. Free monthly email newsletter, *Diabetes Update*, and links to the latest diabetes research.

www.childrenwithdiabetes.com
American website for children, families and adults with diabetes.

www.healthtalk.com/den/
The Diabetes Education Network, a comprehensive source of information about diabetes.

www.diabetesmonitor.com
A resource for patients to educate themselves about their role as active participants in the care of diabetes.

www.diabetesportal.com
A central one-stop resource for people with diabetes and their families.

SUPPLIERS (FOOD)
Aconbury Sprouts
Unit 4, Westwood Industrial Estate, Pontrilas, Hereford HR2 0EL
Tel/fax: 01981 241155
Email: info@aconbury.co.uk
Website: www.aconbury.co.uk
Beansprouts and wheatgrass. Online shopping available through the website.

Allied Bakeries
Vanwall Road, Maidenhead SL6 4UF
Tel: 0870 1121 977
Email: info@burgen.co.uk
Suppliers of Burgen Soy Lin bread.

Aquascot Group Limited
Fyrish Way, Alness, Highlands, Scotland IV17 0PJ
Tel: 01349 884481 Fax: 01349 883893
Email: service@aquascot.uk.com
Website: www.aquascot.com/organic.htm
Wholesale suppliers of organic salmon to Waitrose. Call for stockists.

Bacheldre Watermill
Churchstoke, Montgomery, Powys SY15 6TE
Tel: 01588 620489 Fax: 01588 620105
Email: info@bacheldremill.co.uk
Website: www.bacheldremill.co.uk
Suppliers of excellent quality organic stoneground flour.

Big Oz Industries
PO Box 48, Twickenham,TW1 2UF
Tel: 020 8893 9366 Fax: 020 8893 8799
Email: enquiries@bigoz.co.uk
Website: www.bigoz.co.uk
Organic, gluten-free wholegrain cereals. Call for stockists.

Bioforce (UK) Ltd
2 Brewster Place, Irvine, Scotland KA11 5DD
Tel: 01294 277344 Fax: 01294 277922
Email: enquiries@bioforce.co.uk
Website: www.bioforce.co.uk
Suppliers of BioSnacky bean and seed mixtures for sprouting.

Cauldron Foods Ltd
Units 1-2, Portishead Business Park, Portishead, Bristol BS20 9BF
Tel: 01275 818448
Email: sandrat@cauldronfoods.com
Website: www.cauldronfoods.co.uk
Vegetarian and organic convenience foods, including tofu. Call for stockists.

Clearspring Wholefoods Ltd
19A Acton Park Estate, London W3 7QE
Tel: 020 8749 1781
Website: www.clearspring.co.uk
Organic wholefoods from Japan, including shoyu, tamari and sea vegetables. Online
shopping available through the website.

Coconut Oil UK
PO Box 11045, Dickens Heath, Solihull, West Midlands B90 1ZD
Tel: 0121 744 5753 Fax: 0121 744 5753
Email: info@coconut-oil-uk.com
Website: www.coconut-oil-uk.com
On-line shopping available on the website.

Daily Bread Co-operative
The Old Laundry, Bedford Road, Northampton
Tel: 01604 621531 Fax: 01604 603725
Email: info@dailybread.co.uk
Website: www.dailybread.co.uk
Excellent value wholefood co-operative. Rudimentary online ordering system (orders are sent by email).

Dove's Farm
Salisbury Road, Hungerford, Berkshire RG17 0RF
Tel: 01488 684 880 Fax: 01488 685 235
Email: portenquiry@dovesfarm.co.uk
Website: www.dovesfarm.co.uk
Organic and gluten-free flours, cereals and baked goods. Call for stockists.

Granose Foods Ltd (a division of Haldane Foods)
Howard Way, Newport Pagnell, Bucks MK16 9PY
Tel: 01908 211311 Fax: 01908 210514
Email: info@haldanefoods.co.uk
Website: www.haldanefoods.co.uk
Suppliers of non-hydrogenated margarines and other vegan products. Call for stockists.

Hawkshead Trout Farm
The Boat House, Ridding Wood, Hawkshead, Ambleside, Cumbria LA22 0QF
Tel: 015394 36541 Fax: 015394 36541
Email: trout@hawkshead.demon.co.uk
Website: www.hawskhead.demon.co.uk
Suppliers of organic trout by mail order.

Meridian Foods Ltd
Corwen, Clwyd LL21 9RT
Tel: 01490 413151 Fax: 01490 412032
Email: info@meridianfoods.co.uk
Website: www.meridianfoods.co.uk
Suppliers of organic and special diet foods. Wholesale only. Call for stockists.

Orgran (UK) (Distributors)
Micross, Brent Terrace, London NW2 1LT
Website: www.orgran.com
Australian company supplying gluten-free and wheat-free pastas, crispbreads and snacks.

Sanchi
PO Box 3577, London NW2 1LQ
Shoyu and Tamari soy sauces, sea vegetables, miso, tofu and other Japanese products, available from health food shops.

Seagreens Limited
1 The Warren, Handcross, West Sussex RH17 6DX
Tel: 01444 400403
Fax: 01444 400493
Email: post@seagreens.com
Website: www.seagreens.com
Seaweed granules for cooking and seaweed table condiment. Call for stockists.

Simply Organic Food Company
Horsley Road, Kingsthorpe Hollow, Northampton NN2 6LJ
Tel: 0870 162 3010
Email: info@simplyorganic.net
Website: www.simplyorganic.net
Comprehensive organic mail-order service including fresh foods, groceries, personal
and homecare products.

Suma Wholefoods
Lacy Way, Lowfields Business Park, Elland, West Yorkshire HX5 9DB
Tel: 0845 458 2290 Fax: 0845 458 2295
Email: sales@suma.coop
Website: www.suma.co.uk
Independent wholesaler and distributor of vegetarian, organic and natural foods. Call
for stockists.

Whole Earth Foods Ltd
2 Valentine Place, London SE1 8QH
Tel: 020 7633 5900 Fax: 020 7633 5901
Email: enquiries@wholeearthfoods.co.uk
Website: www.wholeearthfoods.co.uk
Organic drinks, cereals, spread, nut butters. Call for stockists. Online shopping
available on the website.

Woodlands Park Dairy
Woodlands, Wimborne, Dorset BH21 8LX
Tel: 01202 822687 Fax: 01202 826051
Email: info@woodlands-park.co.uk
Website: www.woodlands-park.co.uk
Suppliers of goats and sheeps milk yoghurt.

SUPPLEMENT COMPANIES
The Nutri Centre
7 Park Crescent, London W1N 3HE
Tel: 020 7436 5122 Fax: 020 7436 5171
Website: www.nutricentre.com
The Nutri Centre is situated on the lower ground floor of the Hale Clinic. They are
open to the public and supply a very wide range of supplements from many different
companies as well as an extensive selection of books on nutrition and health. On-line
shopping available on their website.

BioCare Ltd
Lakeside, 180 Lifford Lane, Kings Norton, Birmingham B30 3NU
Tel: 0121 433 3727 Fax: 0121 433 3879
Email: biocare@biocare.co.uk
Website: www.biocare.co.uk
Innovative company originally founded by practitioners for practitioners. Product
range available from The Nutri Centre and selected healthcare stores.

Higher Nature
The Nutrition Centre, Burwash Common, East Sussex TN19 7LX
Tel: 01435 884 668 Fax: 01435 883720
Email: info@higher-nature.co.uk
Website: www.highernature.co.uk
Online shopping available on the website. Product range also available from The
Nutri Centre. Suppliers of Omega organic coconut oil.

REFERENCES

1 Dyson, P. *Nutrition and diabetes control: advice for non-dietitians*. Br J Community Nurs, 2002; 7:414-9.

2 White F, Rafique G. *Diabetes prevalence and projections in South Asia*. Lancet 2002; 360: 07 September 2002.

3 Eschwege, E. *Epidemiology of type II diabetes, diagnosis, prevalence, risk factors, complications*. E.Arch Mal Coeur Vaiss. 2000 Dec; 93 Spec No 4:13-7.

4 Wild, S, Roglic G, Green A, Sicree R, King H. *Global Prevalence of Diabetes: Estimates for the year 2000 and projections for 2030*. Diabetes Care. 2004 May; 27(5):1047-1053.

5 Schernthaner G et al. *Progress in the characterization of slowly progressive autoimmune diabetes in adult patients (LADA or Type 1.5 diabetes)*. Exp Clin Endocrinol Diabetes. 2001;109 Suppl 2:S94-108.

6 Vaarala O, Paronen J, Otonkoski T, Akerblom HK. *Cow milk feeding induces antibodies to insulin in children—a link between cow milk and insulin-dependent diabetes mellitus?* Scand J Immunol. 1998 Feb; 47(2):131-5.

7 Murray M, Pizzorno J, *Textbook of Natural Medicine*, Seattle: John Bastyr College Publications 1988.

8 Given HDC. *A New Angle on Health*. John Bale, Sons & Danielsson Ltd. 1935.

9 Montignac, M. *Dine Out and Lose Weight*. Montignac Publishing (UK) 1996.

10 Willett, W et al. *Glycemic index, glycemic load and risk of Type 2 diabetes*. Am J Clin Nutr 2002;76(suppl):274S-80S.

11 Watts, DL, *Trace Elements and Other Essential Nutrients*, Writer's B-L-O-C-K, 1999.

12 Talior I, Yarkoni M, Bashan N, Eldar-Finkelman H. *Increased glucose uptake promotes oxidative stress and PKC-delta activation in adipocytes of obese, insulin-resistant mice*. Am J Physiol Endocrinol Metab. 2003 Aug; 285(2):E295-302.

13 Bunyard P. *Blowin' in the wind: industrial waste and the government*. The Ecologist 22/6/2001.

14 Reitman et al, Isr. Med Assoc J, 2002, 4; 590-593.

15 Foster-Powell, et al, *International table of glycemic index and glycemic load values: 2002*, Am J Clin Nutr 2002; 76:5-56.

16 Gannon et al, *An increase in dietary protein improves the blood glucose response in persons with Type 2 diabetes*, Am J Clin Nutr. 2003; 78:734-741.

17 Sheela CG, Augusti KT. *Antidiabetic effects of S-allyl cysteine sulphoxide isolated from garlic Allium sativum Linn*. Indian J Exp Biol, 1992; 30: 523-6.

18 Platel K, Srinivasan K. *Plant foods in the management of diabetes mellitus: vegetables as potential hypoglycaemic agents*. Nahrung, 1997; 41:68-74.

19 Madar Z, Stark AH, *New Legume Sources as Therapeutic Agents*, Br J Nutr, 2002; 88:S287-92.

20 Montonen J, Knekt P, Jarvinen R, Reunanen A. *Dietary antioxidant intake and risk of Type 2 diabetes*. Diabetes Care. 2004 Feb; 27(2):362-6.

21 Jiang R et al. *Body iron stores in relation to risk of Type 2 diabetes in apparently healthy women*. JAMA. February 11, 2004;291(6):711-7.

22 Clandinin MT, Wilke MS. *Do trans fatty acids increase the incidence of Type 2 diabetes?* Am J Clin Nutr. June 2001;73:1001-1002, 1019-1026.

23 Fife, Bruce. *The Healing Miracles of Coconut Oil*. Piccadilly Books, 2003.

24 Baba, N. *Enhanced thermogenesis and diminished deposition of fat in response to overfeeding with diet containing medium-chain triglyceride*. Am. J. Clin. Nutr. 1982 35:678

25 Sircar, S. and Kansra, U. 1998. *Choice of cooking oils – myths and realities*. J. Indian Med. Assoc. 96(10):304.

26 Liljeberg H, Bjorck I. *Delayed gastric emptying rate may explain improved glycaemia in healthy subjects to a starchy meal with added vinegar*. Eur J Clin Nutr. 1998 May; 52(5):368-71.

27 Brighenti F et al G. *Effect of neutralized and native vinegar on blood glucose and acetate responses to a mixed meal in healthy subjects*. Eur J Clin Nutr. 1995 Apr; 49(4):242-7.

28 Wien MA et al. *Almonds vs complex carbohydrates in a weight reduction program*. Int J Obes

Metab Disord. 2003 Nov; 27(11): 1365-72.

29 Lopez-Ridaura R et al. *Magnesium intake and risk of Type 2 diabetes in men and women.* Diabetes Care. 2004 Jan; 27(1):134-40.

30 Grylls WK, McKenzie JE, Horwath CC, Mann JI. *Lifestyle factors associated with glycaemic control and body mass index in older adults with diabetes.* Eur J Clin Nutr, 2003:57. 1386-1393.

31 Blaylock, R. *Excito Toxins – The Taste that Kills:* pp39-43, 1997: Health Press, Santa Fe, USA

32 Gregersen S, et al. *Antihyperglycemic effects of stevioside in Type 2 diabetic subjects.* Metabolism 2004; 53(1): 73-76.

33 Keijzers GB, De Galan BE, Tack CJ, Smits P. *Caffeine can decrease insulin sensitivity in humans.* Diabetes Care February 2002;25:364-369.

34 Salazar-Martinez E et al. *Coffee Consumption and Risk for Type 2 Diabetes Mellitus.* Annals of Internal Medicine, 2004; 140:1-8.

35 Rosengren A, Dotevall A, Wilhelmsen L, Thelle D, Johansson S. *Coffee and incidence of diabetes in Swedish women: a prospective 18-year follow-up study.* Intern Med. 2004 Jan; 255(1):89-95.

36 van Dam RM, Feskens EJ. *Coffee consumption and risk of Type 2 diabetes mellitus.* Lancet. 2002 Nov 9;360(9344):1477-8.

37 Howard AA, Arnsten JH, Gourevitch MN. *Effect of alcohol consumption on diabetes mellitus: a systematic review.* Ann Intern Med. 2004 Feb 3;140(3):211-9.

38 Magis DC, Jandrain BJ, Scheen AJ. *Alcohol, insulin sensitivity and diabetes.* Rev Med Liège. 2003 Jul-Aug; 58(7-8):501-7.

39 Bell DS. *Alcohol and the NIDDM patient.* Diabetes Care. 1996 May; 19(5):509-13.

40 Wannamethee SG et al. *Alcohol drinking patterns and risk of Type 2 diabetes mellitus among younger women.* Arch Intern Med. 2003 Jun 9;163(11):1329-36.

41 Ames RP. *The effect of sodium supplementation on glucose tolerance and insulin concentrations in patients with hypertension and diabetes mellitus.* American Journal of Hypertension, 2001, Vol 14, Iss 7, Part 1, pp 653-659.

42 Khan A, Safdar M, Ali Khan MM, Khattak KN, Anderson RA. *Cinnamon improves glucose and lipids of people with Type 2 diabetes.* Diabetes Care 26:3215-3218, 2003.

43 Barringer TA, Kirk JK, Santaniello AC, Foley KL, Michielutte R. *Effect of a multivitamin and mineral supplement on infection and quality of life.* A randomized, double-blind, placebo-controlled trial. Ann Intern Med 2003; 138(5):365-71.

44 Block G et al. *Plasma C-reactive protein concentrations in active and passive smokers: influence of antioxidant supplementation.* J Am Coll Nutr 2004 Apr; 23(2):141-7.

45 Timms PM et al. *Circulating MMP9, vitamin D and variation in the TIMP-1 response with VDR genotype: mechanisms for inflammatory damage in chronic disorders?* QJM. 2002 Dec; 95(12):787-96.

46 Hypponen E, Laara E, Reunanen A. *Intake of vitamin D and risk of Type 1 diabetes: a birth-cohort study.* Lancet. 2001 Nov 3;358(9292):1500-3.

47 Ortlepp JR, Lauscher J, Hoffmann R. *The vitamin D receptor gene variant is associated with the prevalence of Type 2 diabetes mellitus and coronary artery disease.* Diabet Med. 2001 Oct; 18(10):842-5.

48 Quillot D et al. *Fatty acid abnormalities in chronic pancreatitis: effect of concomitant diabetes mellitus.* Eur J Clin Nutr 57(3): 496-503, Mar 2003.

49 Annual Experimental Biology 2002 Conference New Orleans, LA April 21, 2002.

50 Petersen M et al. *Effect of fish oil versus corn oil supplementation on LDL and HDL subclasses in Type 2 diabetic patients.* Diabetes Care October 2002;25:1704-1708.

51 Ma J et al. *Associations of serum and dietary magnesium with cardiovascular disease, hypertension, diabetes, insulin, and carotid arterial wall thickness: the ARIC study.* Atherosclerosis Risk in Communities Study. J Clin Epidemiol. 1995 Jul; 48(7):927-40.

52 Arvanitakis Z, Wilson RS, Bienias JL, Evans DA, Bennett DA. *Diabetes mellitus and risk of Alzheimer disease and decline in cognitive function.* Arch Neurol. 2004 May; 61(5):661-6.

53 www.tahoma-clinic.com.

54 Mooradian AD et al. *Selected vitamins and minerals in diabetes.* Diabetes Care 1994 May; 17(5):464-79.

55 Ghosh D et al. *Role of chromium supplementation in Indians with Type 2 diabetes mellitus.* J

Nutr Biochem. 2002 Nov; 13(11):690-697.

56 Ambrosch A et al. *Relation between homocysteinaemia and diabetic neuropathy in patients with Type 2 diabetes mellitus.* Diabet Med. 2001 Mar; 18(3):185-92.

57 Liu X, Zhou HJ, Rohdewald P. *French maritime pine bark extract Pycnogenol dose-dependently lowers glucose in Type 2 diabetic patients.* Diabetes Care. 2004 Mar; 27(3):839.

58 Sotaniemi EA, Haapakoski E, Rautio A. *Ginseng therapy in non-insulin-dependent diabetic patients.* Diabetes Care 1995 Oct; 18(10):1373-5.

59 Leatherdale BA et al. *Improvement in glucose tolerance due to Momordica charantia (karela).* Br Med J (Clin Res Ed). 1981 Jun 6;282(6279):1823-4.

60 Baskaran K et al. *Antidiabetic effect of a leaf extract from Gymnema sylvestre in non-insulin-dependent diabetes mellitus patients.* J Ethnopharmacol. 1990 Oct; 30(3):295-300.

61 Jia W, Gao W, Tang L. *Antidiabetic herbal drugs officially approved in China.* Phytother Res. 2003 Dec; 17(10):1127-34.

62 Wannamethee SG, Shaper AG, Alberti KG. *Physical activity, metabolic factors, and the incidence of coronary heart disease and Type 2 diabetes.* Arch Intern Med. 2000 Jul 24;160(14):2108-16.

63 Surwit RS et al. *Stress management improves long-term glycaemic control in Type 2 diabetes.* Diabetes Care. 2002 Jan; 25(1):30-4.

64 Wang Q. *The present situation of TCM treatment for diabetes and its researches.* J Tradit Chin Med. 2003 Mar; 23(1):67-73.

65 Galper DI, Taylor AG, Cox DJ. *Current status of mind-body interventions for vascular complications of diabetes.* Family and Community Health 26(1): 34-40, Jan-Mar 2003.

66 Ayas NT et al. *A prospective study of self-reported sleep duration and incident diabetes in women.* Diabetes Care. 2003 Feb; 26(2):380-4.

67 Hooper PL. *Hot-tub therapy for Type 2 diabetes mellitus.* N Engl J Med, 1999; 341: 924-5.

68 Hayashi K et al. *Laughter lowered the increase in postprandial blood glucose.* Diabetes Care May 2003;26:1651-1652.

69 Arch Intern Med, 2000; 160:1009-13.

70 Madar Z, Stark AH. *New Legume Sources as Therapeutic Agents,* Br J Nutr, 2002; 88:S287-92.

71 Swanston-Flatt SK, Day C, Bailey CJ, Flatt PR. *Traditional plant treatments for diabetes. Studies in normal and streptozotocin diabetic mice.* Diabetologia. 1990 Aug; 33(8):462-4.

INDEX

NOTES

NOTES